THE MODERN
APOTHECARY

An Hachette UK Company
www.hachette.co.uk

First published in Great Britain in 2024 by
Kyle Books, an imprint of Octopus Publishing Group Limited
Carmelite House
50 Victoria Embankment
London EC4Y 0DZ
www.octopusbooks.co.uk

ISBN: 9781804191408

Distributed in the US by Hachette Book Group, 1290 Avenue of the Americas, 4th and 5th Floors, New York, NY 10104

Distributed in Canada by Canadian Manda Group, 664 Annette St., Toronto, Ontario, Canada M6S 2C8

Printed and bound in China

10 9 8 7 6 5 4 3 2 1

FSC MIX
Paper | Supporting responsible forestry
FSC® C008047

Publisher: Joanna Copestick
Project Editor: Samhita Foria
Art Director: Juliette Norsworthy
Design: Rachel Cross
Production: Lisa Pinnell
Photography: Sam Scales
Illustration: Kate Straughan

anatomē

THE MODERN APOTHECARY

How to harness the
power of botanicals to
support your health
and improve wellbeing

BRENDAN MURDOCK

GABRIEL WEIL

KYLE BOOKS

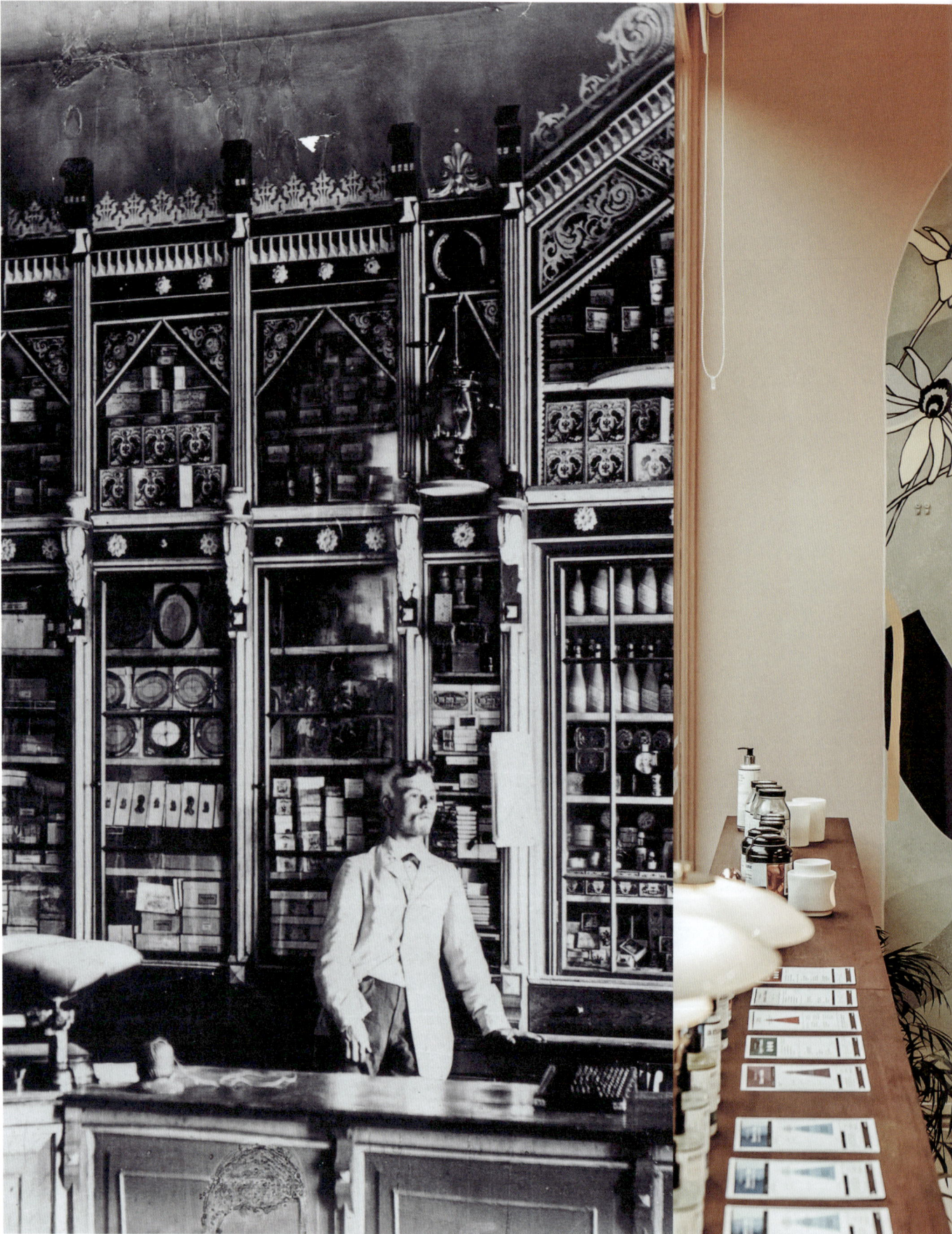

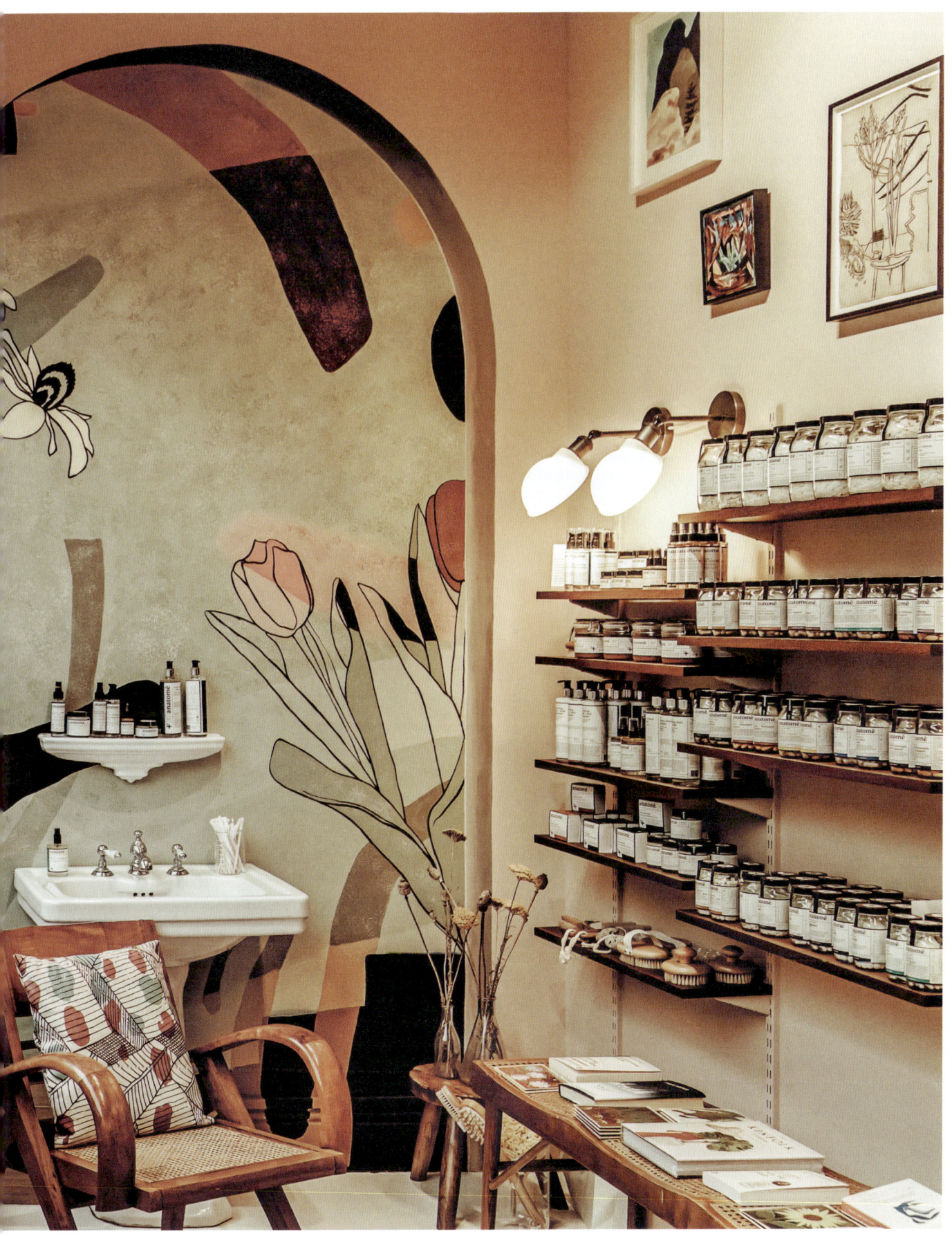

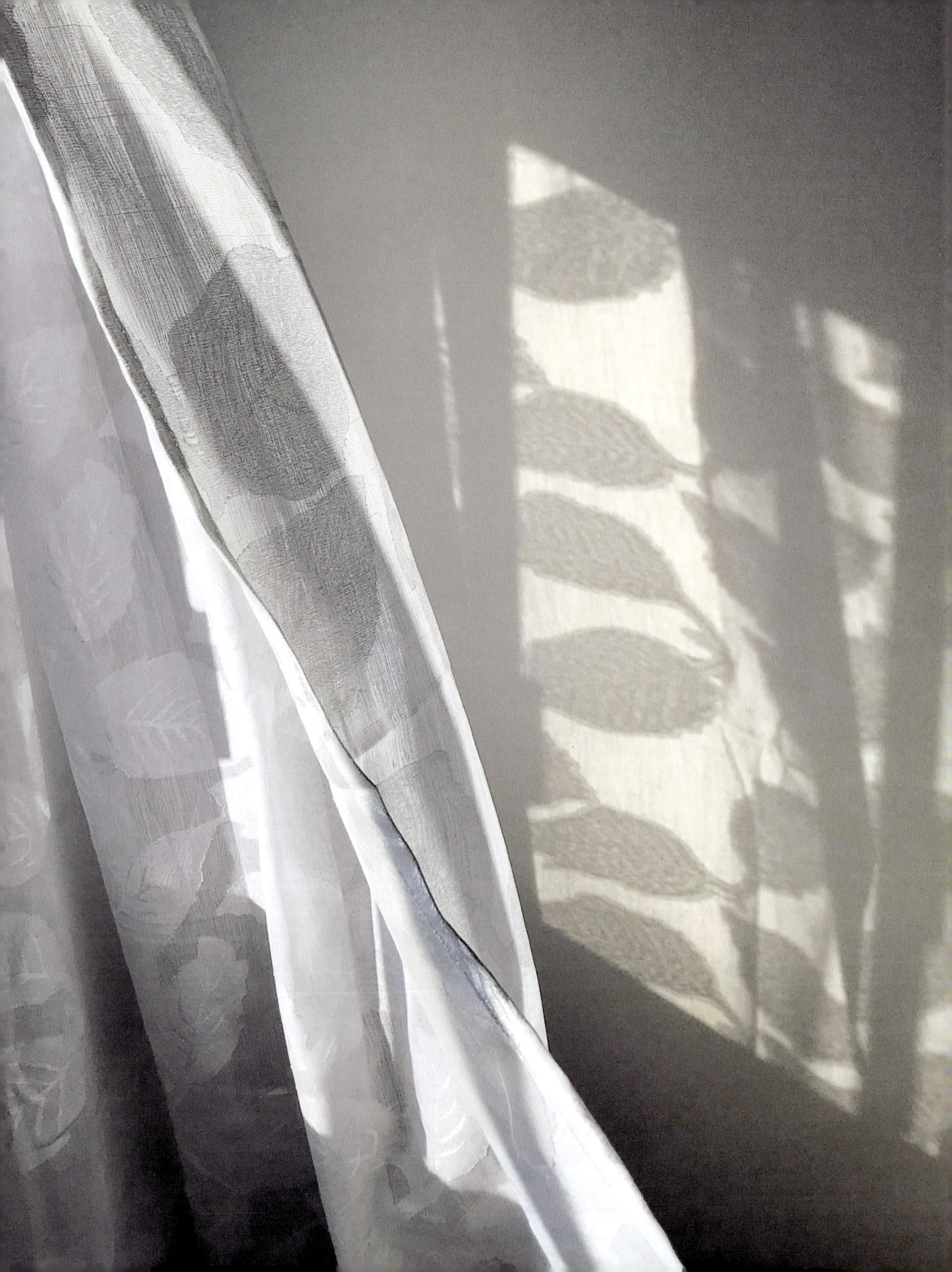

CONTENTS

Introduction **8**

WELLBEING THROUGH TIME
How are you today? **12**
Wellbeing – a positive cycle **16**
Wellbeing through the ages **20**

THE APOTHECARY
A spicer, a grocer and a pharmacist **28**
Branding wellbeing through the ages **32**
anatomē: London's modern apothecary **36**
What is aromachology? **40**

WELLBEING PILLARS
Today's wellbeing yearnings **46**
1. Sleep **48**
   Sleep through the ages **58**
2. Balance **62**
3. Movement **70**
   Exercise through the ages **80**
4. Focus **84**
5. Diet **96**
   Diets through the ages **98**
Wellbeing villains **106**

WELLBEING PRACTICES
What are wellbeing practices? **126**
Sleep practice **136**
Bathroom practice **142**
Create your haven **146**
Meditate **150**
Massage **158**
Get outdoors **160**

HERO BOTANICALS
The power of botanicals **166**

Further reading **220**
Index **221**
Acknowledgements **223**
About the authors **224**

INTRODUCTION

Wellness isn't a new concept. Humanity's quest for wellbeing has been consistent throughout history, spanning civilizations and cultures. From the ancient Egyptians' belief in the balance of mind, body and soul to the teachings of Greek philosophers such as Hippocrates emphasizing holistic health, we find evidence of early pursuits of wellbeing that still serve as a reference in modern medicine.

Eastern traditions, such as Ayurveda and traditional Chinese medicine, offer comprehensive systems promoting harmony and vitality. As centuries progressed, the Renaissance sparked a renewed interest in physical and mental wellbeing, with the likes of Leonardo da Vinci studying anatomy and pursuing holistic health practices.

Apothecaries and health purveyors have played an important role in wellbeing history, evolving from ancient civilizations where merchants traded spices, herbs and remedies. Over time, they transformed into esteemed establishments offering medicinal compounds, advice and healthcare services.

Humanity evolves, but our basic wellbeing needs remain: this enduring pursuit continues as we explore innovative approaches that integrate ancient wisdom with modern scientific advancements to nurture our wellbeing.

That's why anatomē was born: to bridge health and lifestyle, bringing life-enhancing practices and formulations to communities and helping people look after themselves. To recreate the apothecary experience in an era of scientific knowledge, losing the witchcraft connotations and maintaining the trustworthy aspect of the community merchant with solutions to people's needs.

Moreover, anatomē brings a new answer to consumer lifestyle cravings: viewing wellbeing as the ultimate luxury – more valuable than any other status symbol. You'll wear your wellbeing better than any new watch or handbag.

This book explores the history and ingredients in our formulations, recipes, practices, anecdotes and the knowledge behind our brand and philosophy. It gives readers a glimpse into aromachology – the science that studies how scent can support our body functioning and provides comprehensive guidance on how to incorporate this science and harness its benefits to enhance busy, dynamic lifestyles.

Rather than establish rules or increase anxiety around how we feel, this book highlights simple ways to improve everyday life with easy-to-follow practices and practical ways of incorporating powerful botanical ingredients to help us feel better.

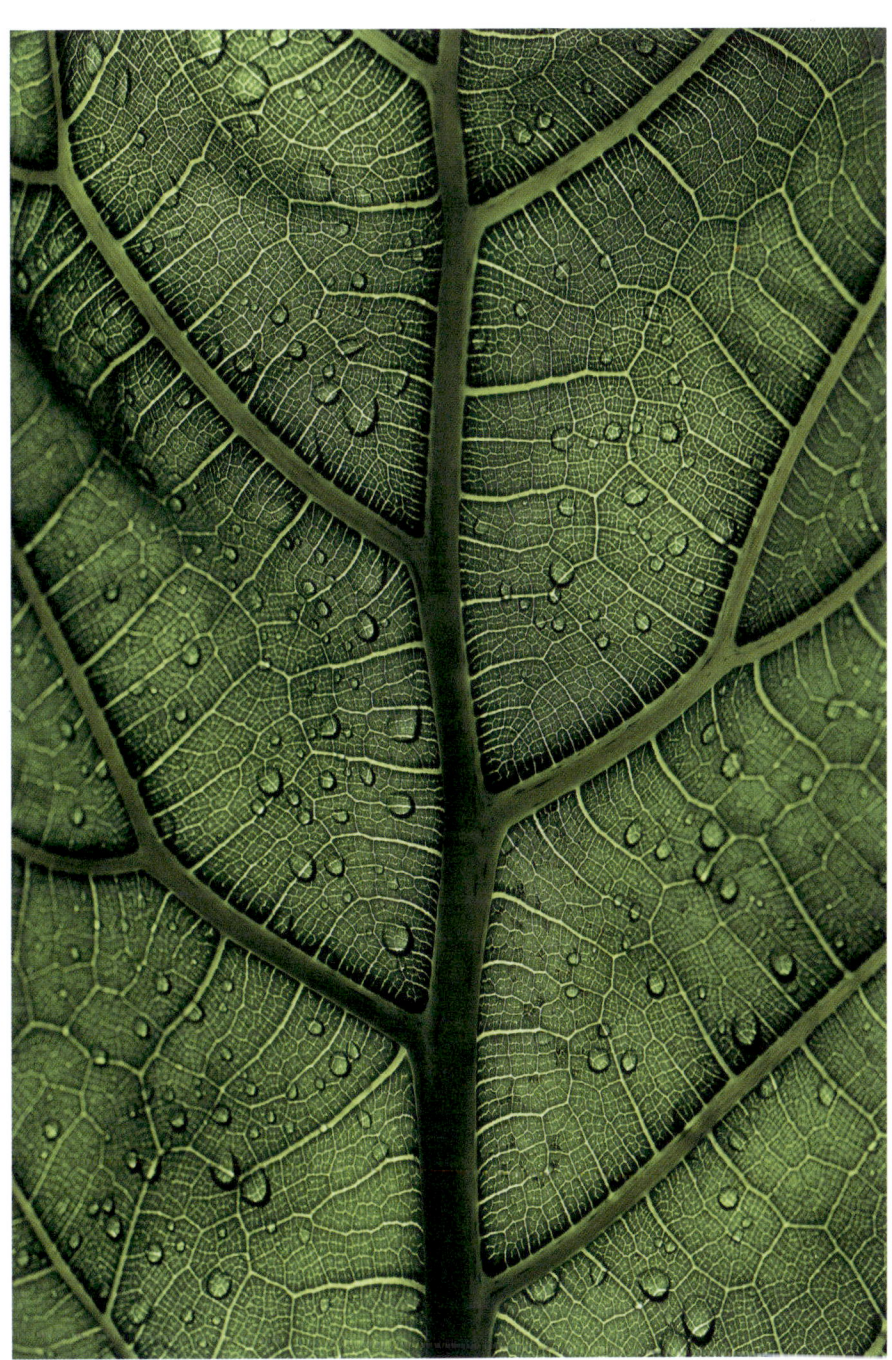

WEL
TH

LBEING

ROUGH

TIME

HOW
ARE
YOU
TODAY

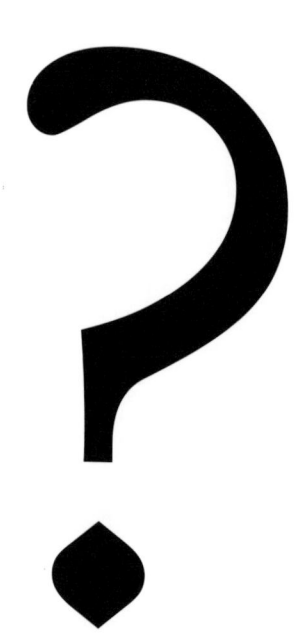

If you left your home today and interacted with a human being or two, you likely asked them how they were doing. And you were probably asked the same, either in return or as an opener.

When did showing interest in another person's wellbeing become a form of social etiquette?

'How do you do?' 'How do you fare?' These and other how-do sentences can be traced back to the 1370s, mostly in plays, as official documents are less likely to register this colloquial form of language.

As far as research goes, however, the specific question 'How are you?' wasn't recorded, at least in writing, until the 1600s. The record in question is an exchange in Thomas Middleton's play *Women Beware Women* (c. 1621):

'How are you now, sir?'
'I feel a better ease, madam.'

Today, as societies grow increasingly self-centred, even the politest replies of 'I'm well, thank you', can annoy the interlocutor. There's no need to ask it back either: no one wants to know.

But we do want to know how we are feeling. And we want to talk about it, too. The truthful answers, positive or negative, reveal our wellbeing yearnings. And we all have them.

anatomē's aim is to create a culture, a conversation, where our community can discuss their wellbeing needs and challenges with a team prepared to address them. This book is a curated selection of this information, with anecdotal and science-backed facts that will help you embrace health and wellbeing from a preventative perspective.

Sleep, focus, movement, balance and gut health aren't health emergencies, but lingering subjects we avoid or ignore while we get on with our days. Often results of careless routines and not-so-great habits, these challenges can be faced with practices, natural ingredients and a welcome dose of awareness.

After reading this book, you will probably need to keep your polite 'I'm doing well, thank you'. But, with manageable lifestyle changes, you'll master 'I could have slept better', or 'I am struggling to concentrate'. Most of all, after this journey of revisiting wellbeing from the past and interacting with it in the present, we want you to be more aware of what equilibrium means for you, what foods work for you, how many hours sleep is enough, your own moods and the practices you need to adopt so you can live, and live well, to be well.

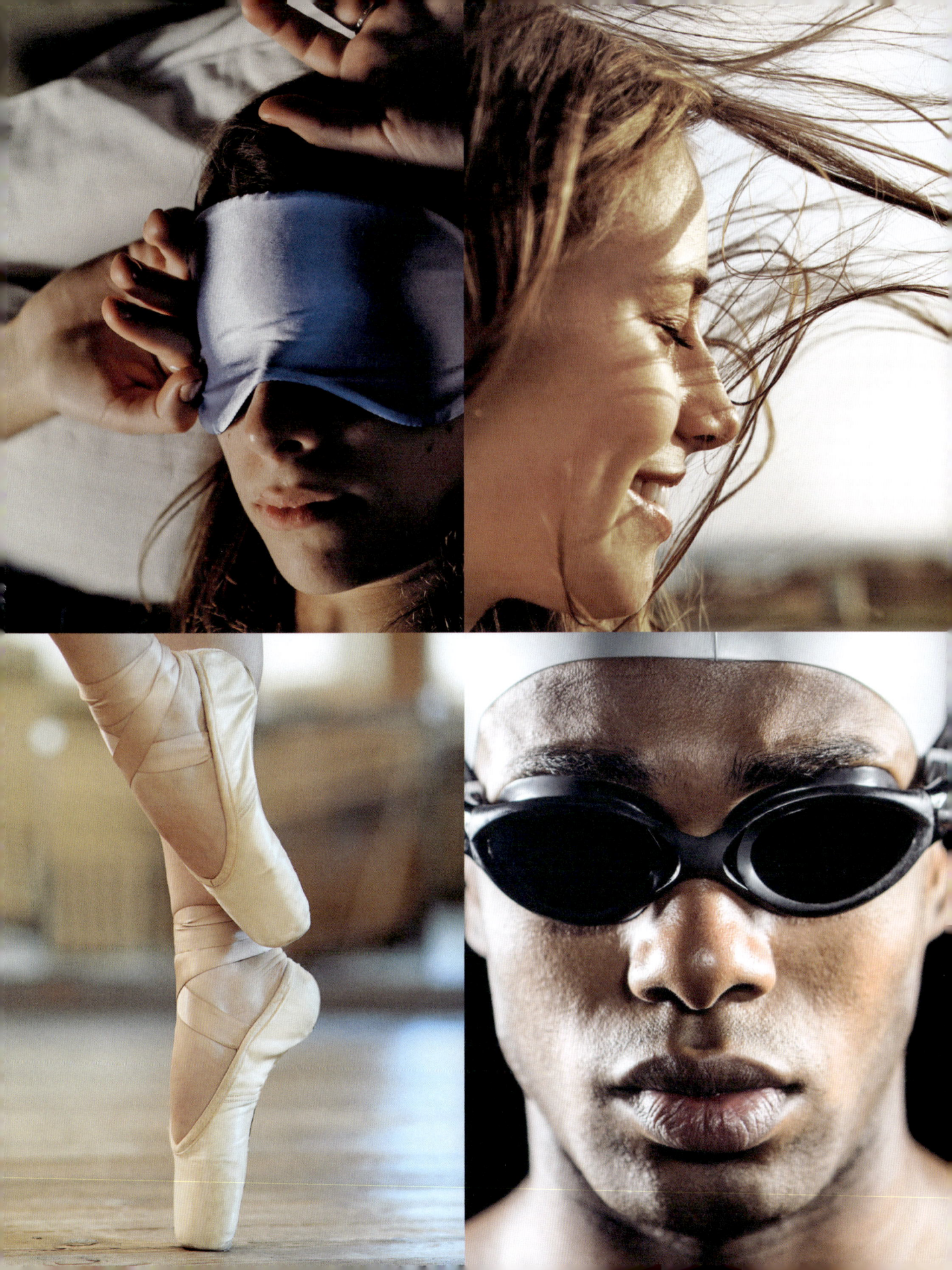

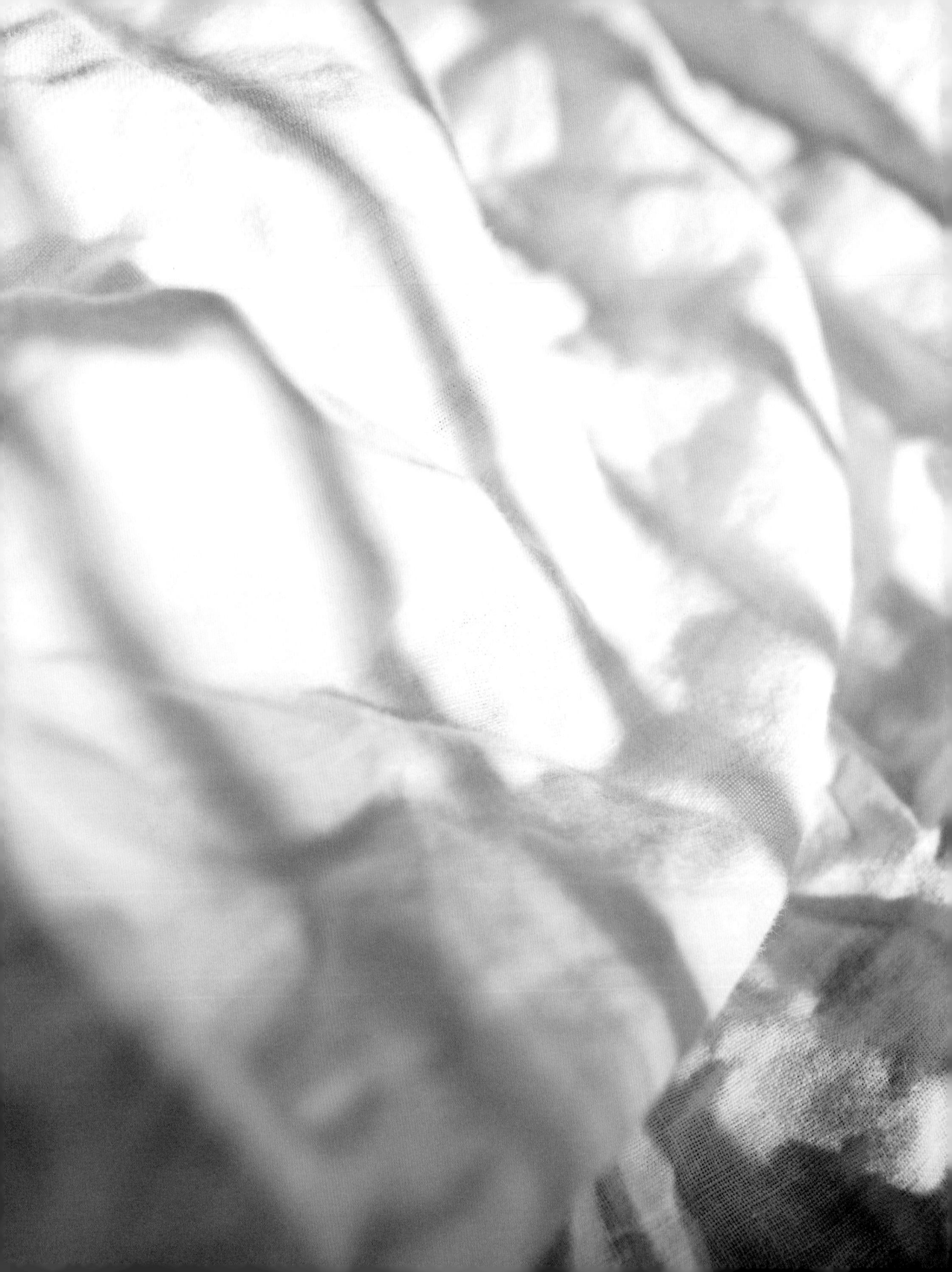

WELLBEING –
A POSTIVE CYCLE

The term wellbeing refers to being comfortable, happy and
in good health. It can refer to an entire society, our planet,
a nation or an individual.

We can interpret wellbeing in many ways. Someone saving money may be thinking about their future wellbeing (secured with financial backing). A government may be concerned about social wellbeing and taking social measures to ensure people are well.

The Centers for Disease Control and Prevention (CDC) in the US defines wellbeing as an overall perception that life is going well. The level of this measure can start with the basics, such as housing, employment and nourishment. It then evolves and changes meaning depending on the demographics analyzed.

WHAT IS WELLBEING?

For someone with a job, appropriate housing and a lifestyle where all their living needs are met, the definition of wellbeing applies to their mental and physical health.

We will look at the anatomē community as a demographic with a comfortable lifestyle. Financially stable and provided with all their basic needs, plus their luxury of choice (with the idea of luxury varying from one individual to another). That may seem an obvious observation, but understanding the relativity of wellbeing ensures we're not insensitive to societal problems. Addressing the sleep quality of someone with a heated home, quality food and a comfortable lifestyle is different from addressing the needs of people without a home or someone unemployed facing financial difficulties.

LINK TO HEALTH

At anatomē, we see wellbeing as a positive cycle we can generate and nurture. It involves everyday health aspects often ignored or overlooked, such as the quality of our sleep, disposition, energy and focus.

Wellbeing manifestations – as well as symptoms from lack of wellbeing – are linked. Once you tackle one aspect of your wellbeing, you'll likely notice improvements in other areas of your life too.

We will discuss some wellbeing aspects in depth, addressing the subjects we've mastered with our research. We will also gently discuss some of the repercussions of a successful regimen of wellbeing practices. For example, someone with improved sleep quality will likely enjoy sex more.

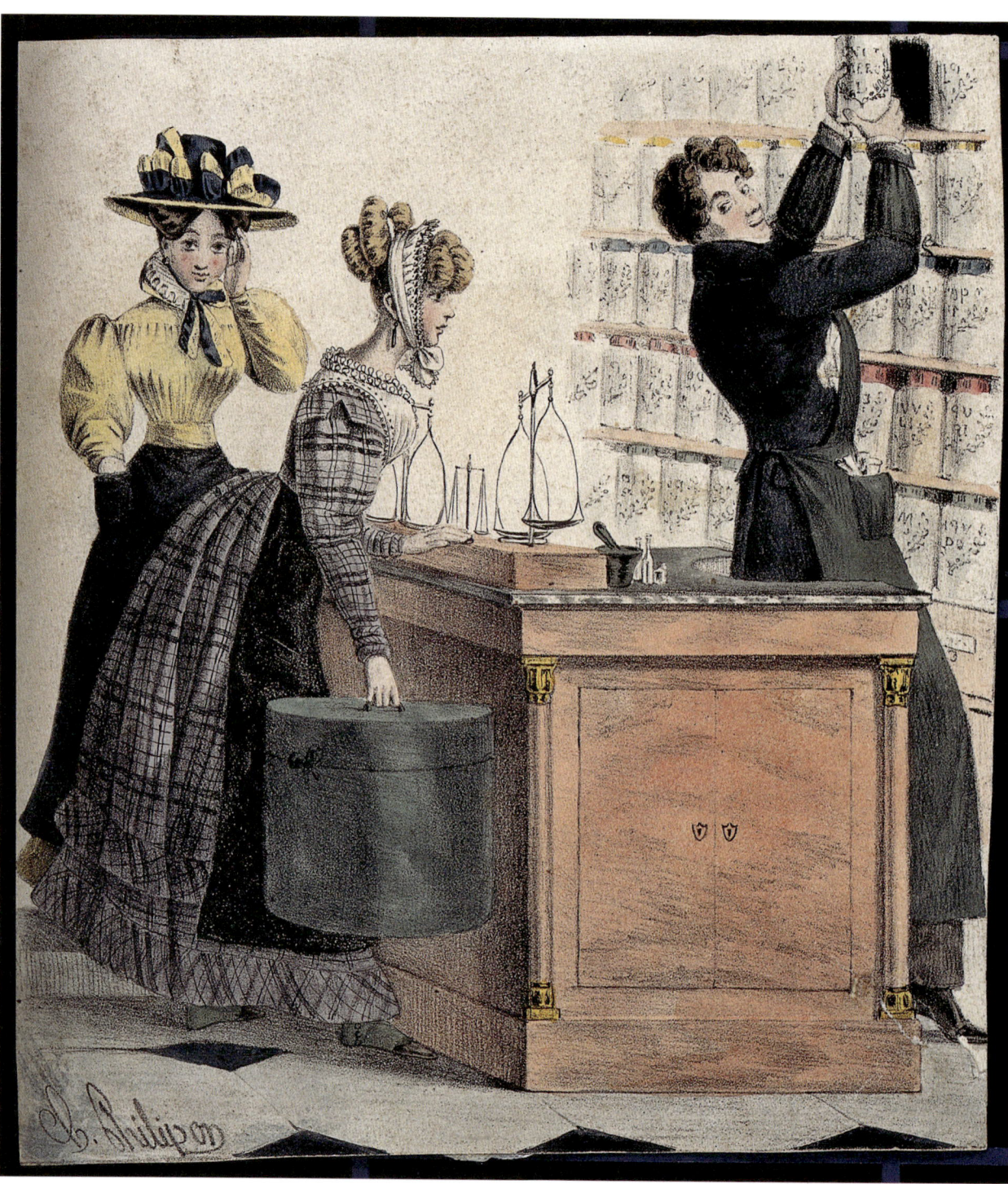

Each wellbeing aspect we tackle at anatomē comes with a list of 'halo-effect' improvements. These are benefits that go beyond the initial challenge and improve many aspects of life, thanks to our increased resilience, better physical health, improved cognitive function and greater life satisfaction.

Once you tackle one aspect of your wellbeing, you'll likely notice improvements in other areas of your life too.

WELLNESS: AN ANCIENT CONCEPT

Wellbeing originates from wellness, a modern concept with ancient roots. We only began to discuss and understand wellness as we do today in the mid-twentieth century.

What changed is the rapid development of the perception of an individual and their psychological and physical state. Also during this period, the idea of 'healthy habits' and preventing illnesses became mainstream. Rather than being 'healthy' or 'ill', today we assess our health risks, we have routine checks and we're learning to talk about ourselves and our mental health.

We also take a more nuanced (less black-and-white) approach to how we feel. There's a broad spectrum of health and wellness levels – all relative and individual. While your medical exams may show overall good health, your self-care may need a switch to make you feel at ease.

Being healthy is also about our daily paths. Drinking more water, taking an outdoor walk, meditating and practising awareness, improving your sleep, managing your diet, feeling focused and present: how do you keep your health in check day-to-day?

WELLBEING THROUGH THE AGES

Wellbeing, as a concept, has existed for a long time. While civilizations have always sought ways to improve their health, the understanding of wellness has evolved and changed with time. Understanding the breakthroughs of wellbeing through the centuries, medicine's oscillating approach between cure and prevention of illnesses and the advent of wellness beyond physical health helps us understand the present.

3,000– 1,500 BC

Ayurveda is a holistic health and wellness system of practices and formulations that strives to create harmony between body, mind and spirit. Ayurvedic regimens are tailored to the individual's constitution, including their nutritional, exercise, social and hygiene needs – aiming to create a physical and mental balance that prevents illness. Among Ayurvedic practices now widely used are yoga and meditation.

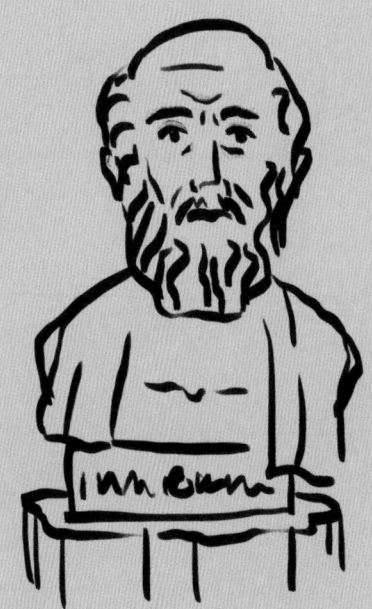

500 BC

In ancient Greece, Hippocrates was arguably the pioneering physician to propose preventative medicine. He believed in working against sickness before it happened over treating diseases. Hippocrates was also the first physician to state that health problems can be consequences of diet, lifestyle and environmental factors, such as air quality, water purity, climate and sanitation.

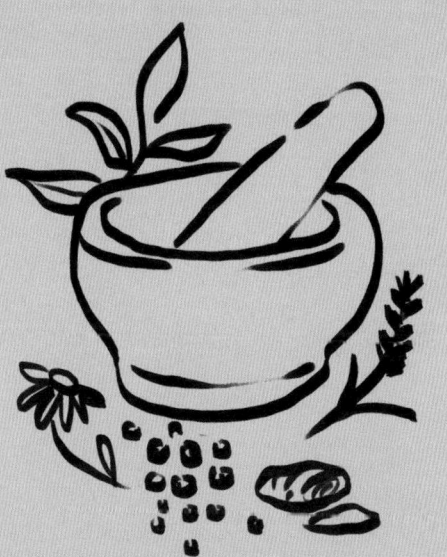

50 BC

In ancient Rome, medicine was highly preventative – based on the Greek philosophy – focusing on the individual's diet and lifestyle. Romans also had a highly developed public health system and public infrastructure. With aqueducts, sewers and public baths, their high hygiene standards prevented the spread of infections and earned them a healthier population.

200–300 AD

Historical records of women in medicine are rare, as are studies focusing solely on women's health. In *On the Diseases and Cures of Women*, Metrodora wrote about conditions affecting the uterus, abdomen and kidneys, fertility treatments and even shares recipes for contraception.

1730s

The plates of *A Curious Herbal*, published between 1737 and 1739, were illustrated and engraved by the Scottish botanist and author Elizabeth Blackwell. The book featured illustrations of medicinal plants and was created as a resource for pharmacists and doctors.

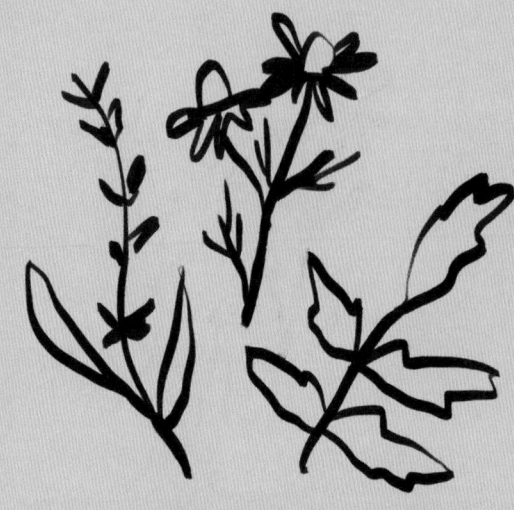

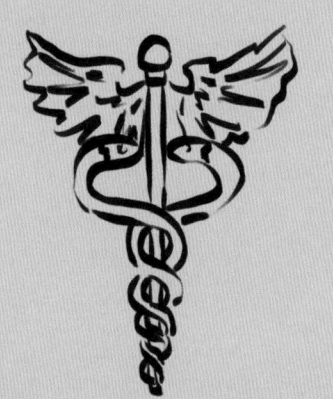

1650s

Wellness becomes a word in the English language. In the earliest published reference, dating from 1654, this term referred to the antonym of 'illness'. The record in question was a diary entry of Sir Archibald Johnston: '*I ... blessed God ... for my daughter's wealnesse.*'

The Oxford English Dictionary dates this expression to this decade. This term, however, referred to more than simply 'not being ill', but to 'the state of being healthy, especially when you actively try to achieve this'.

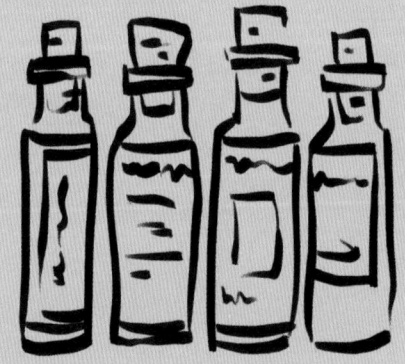

1790s

Homeopathy appears in Germany. Physician Samuel Hahnemann led the development of a health system utilizing natural substances to promote self-healing responses from the body. Homeopaths, a category of 200,000 physicians in practice today, believe in curing sick people with substances that cause symptoms of a given disease in those who are healthy.

1870s

Osteopathy, a holistic system based on the manipulation of muscles and joints developed by Andrew Taylor Still develops. In modern medicine, osteopathy is a speciality practised by nearly 200,000 physicians.

1880s

Chiropractic is born. American chiropractor Daniel David Palmer manipulated the back of janitor Harvey Lillard, readjusting bones and joints and discovering a way to mechanically fix the skeleton. Today, chiropractic is a recognized alternative, complementary type of medicine.

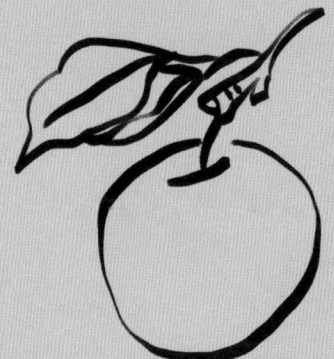

1860s

Also in Germany, a Catholic priest named Sebastian Kneipp introduced his eponymous cure system. Naming it 'Kneipp Cure', he combined herbalism, hydrotherapy and a regime of exercise and nutrition to treat and prevent disease.

Also during this period, the first recorded movement of cure promoted by a healthy mind appeared: *Theories of Mentally Aided Healing* by Phineas Parkhurst Quimby.

1890s

Nutritional research is at the heart of the work of Swiss physician Maximilian Bircher-Benner. He advocates a diet with higher, consistent portions of fruits and vegetables to keep an individual healthy, holistically protecting bodily functions.

1900s

John Harvey Kellogg, director of Battle Creek Sanitarium in Michigan, advocates an early version of what we today understand as a healthy, wholesome lifestyle. Naturopathy consists of exercise, fresh air, a healthy diet and hydrotherapy, composing an overall notion of 'learning to be well'. This system was supported by herbal formulations, massages and other wellbeing practices – close to anatomē's practices.

In Austria, Rudolf Steiner, a philosopher interested in spirituality, develops the anthroposophy movement, which emphasized the spiritual nature of humanity, and anthroposophical holistic medicine, an approach that sought to treat the whole individual, including their physical, emotional and spiritual needs.

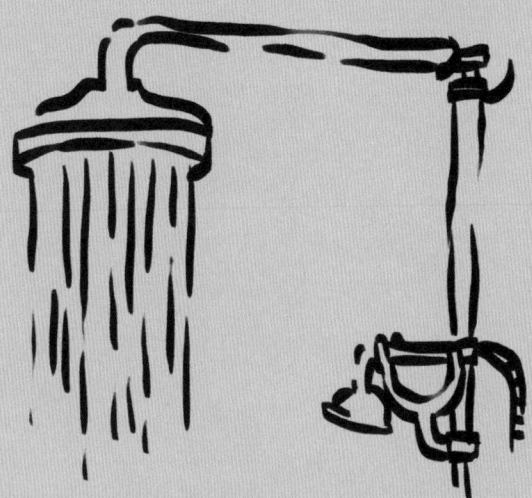

1960s

Chinese pharmaceutical chemist, and malariologist, Tu Youyou discovers artemisinin and dihydroartemisinin, compounds used to treat malaria, by reading traditional Chinese medical texts. This breakthrough has helped save millions of lives in South China, Southeast Asia, Africa and South America.

1950s

Wellness gets its modern meaning. The pioneering concept appears in a work by Halbert L. Dunn called *High-Level Wellness* (published in 1961). Dr Dunn was one of the first physicians to broaden the understanding of wellness by recognizing alternatives to evidence-driven, disease-focused biomedicine, which was then the only recognized form of health treatment. He assembles studies, practices and beliefs to develop the idea of wellness, which was abstract at the time. From this moment, a series of movements would defend wellness as a holistic societal challenge, as well as something that could be fostered with public policies on everything from farming to pollution control, and later to mental health management and support.

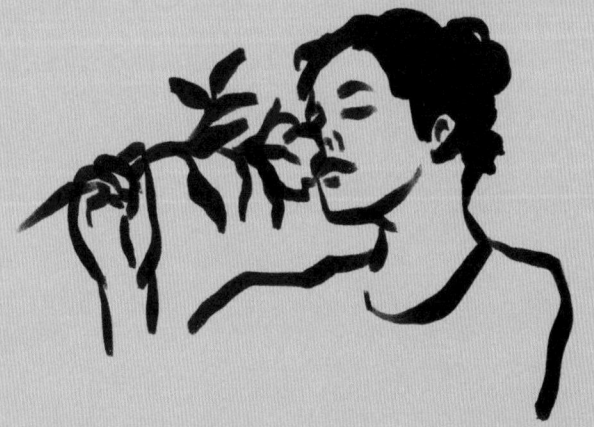

1980s

The wellness movement is taken seriously by corporations, medical organizations and academia. One of the most prominent publications of this movement was the *Berkeley Wellness Letter*, which began in 1984. It presented science-backed articles, often contradicting medical beliefs, gaining momentum and followers.

Actress and activist Jane Fonda launched *Jane Fonda's Workout* in 1982, an exercise routine on video, launched with a focus on helping women exercise at home. The VHS tape became a bestseller and led to a movement of celebrity-endorsed wellbeing practices and guides, still in vogue today.

Also during this period, wellness reached the mainstream as a new industry, with fitness programmes, workplace awareness and celebrity-created and endorsed products and brands.

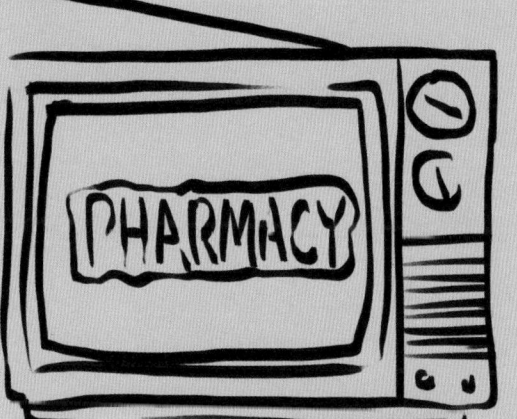

2010s

The advent of social media allowed audiences to publish their ideas. First in images, then through videos, a growing number of individuals share their wellbeing practices, including diet, skincare, exercise and haven-creation on social media. Known as influencers, they achieve global success and recognition and reach celebrity status, shifting perceptions of trust and research and focusing on individual experiences and stories.

APOTH

THE
ECARY

A SPICER, A GROCER AND A PHARMACIST

The 'apotheca' was the Roman name given to a storage area for spices, wines, spirits and herbs. In thirteenth-century England, the commerçants holding stock of such goods received a title in society: the apothecary. From Vienna to Washington every main street had an apothecary.

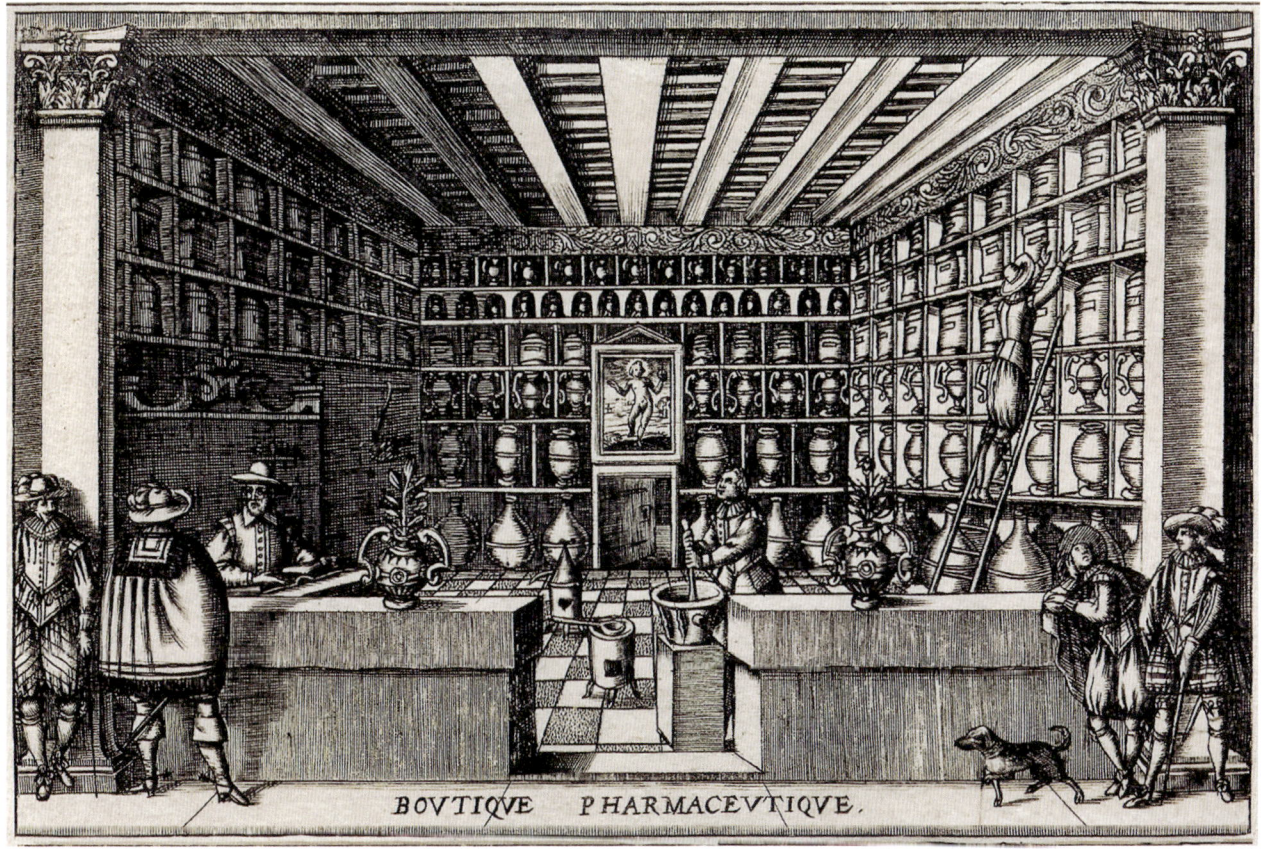

BOVTIQVE PHARMACEVTIQVE.

Apothecaries had a shop or stall, as grocers did. But their speciality, non-staple goods, earned them a distinctive classification. Before this denomination, these tradesmen were known as pepperers or spicers.

Over time, apothecaries expanded their selection of goods with medicinal herbs, perfumes, confectionery and drugs, as well as preparations they created and sold to the public, promising health, mood and quality-of-life improvements.

Fast forward to the mid-sixteenth century, and the apothecary trade had evolved into the equivalent of modern pharmacies. The focus of this trade was mainly medicinal, although medicinal practices continued to be regulated the Royal College of Physicians (RCP), a professional body that sets standards for physicians and promotes the study of medicine.

On 6 December 1617, after a petition led by apothecary Gideon de Laune, whose patients (or customers) included Anne of Denmark, the wife of James I, the Worshipful Society of Apothecaries of London was incorporated by royal charter.

King James, at the time, made a statement defending the trade: 'I myself did devise that corporation and do allow it. The grocers, who complain of it, are but merchants; the mystery of these apothecaries were belonging to apothecaries, wherein the grocers are unskilful; and therefore I think it is fitting they should be a corporation of themselves.'

In 1673, the Society of Apothecaries founded the Chelsea Physic Garden as a teaching garden for apothecaries to study and cultivate medicinal plants to produce various formulations, such as tinctures, ointments and syrups. These formulations were used to treat a wide range of ailments and diseases, including respiratory disorders, digestive issues, skin conditions and more. The garden also served as a resource for medical research and education, and has been visited by many notable physicians and botanists wishing to study its plants and their medicinal properties.

Today, the Chelsea Physic Garden continues to serve as a valuable resource for education, conservation and research in the field of herbal medicine.

The history of apothecaries has a series of losses and wins in maintaining its recognition. With the rise of the pharmaceutical industry, the role of apothecaries has evolved, and they now primarily work in the community pharmacy setting. Outside of the UK, the term 'apothecary' is not commonly used, and the community pharmacist's role varies depending on the country's healthcare system.

In India, traditional Ayurvedic practitioners serve as apothecaries, preparing and dispensing herbal remedies to treat a range of ailments, while in the Middle East, traditional herbal medicine is still practised, with some practitioners serving as apothecaries by preparing and dispensing herbal remedies to treat various health conditions.

anatomē
Cornish Lavender
Scented Candle
Bougie Parfumée
anatomē
Bath & Shower Oil
Huile de bain et douche
Roman Chamomile
anatomē
Overactive Mind
anatomē
Pillow Spray
Vaporisateur d'oreiller
Somali Frankincense
anatomē
Bath & Shower Oil
Huile de bain et douche
Cornish Lavender
anatomē
Stressed Mind
anatomē
Pillow Spray
Vaporisateur d'oreiller
Roman Chamomile
anatomē
Bath & Shower Oil
Huile de bain et douche
Somali Frankincense
anatomē
Restless Mind
anatomē
Somali Frankincense
Scented Candle
Bougie Parfumée

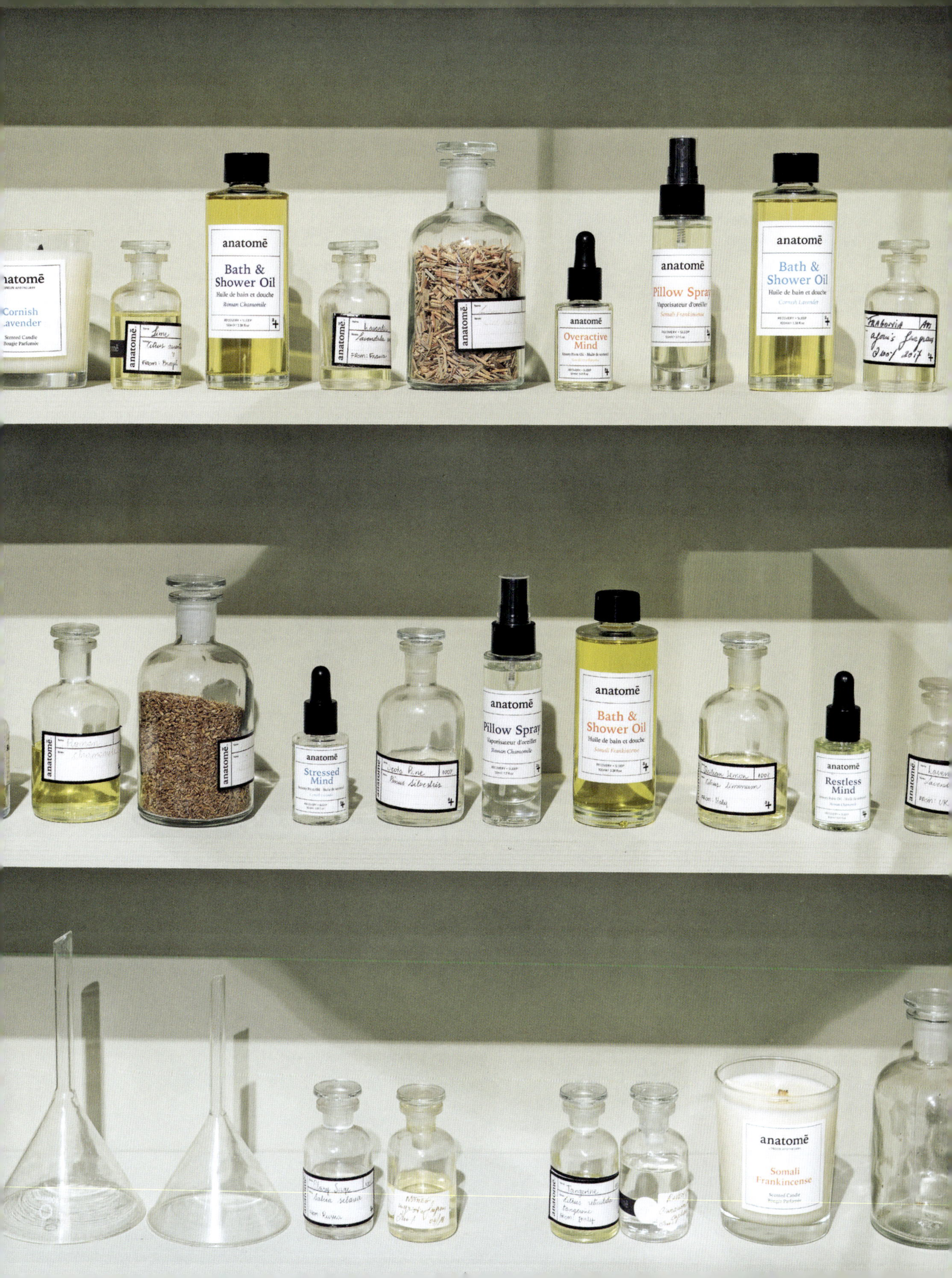

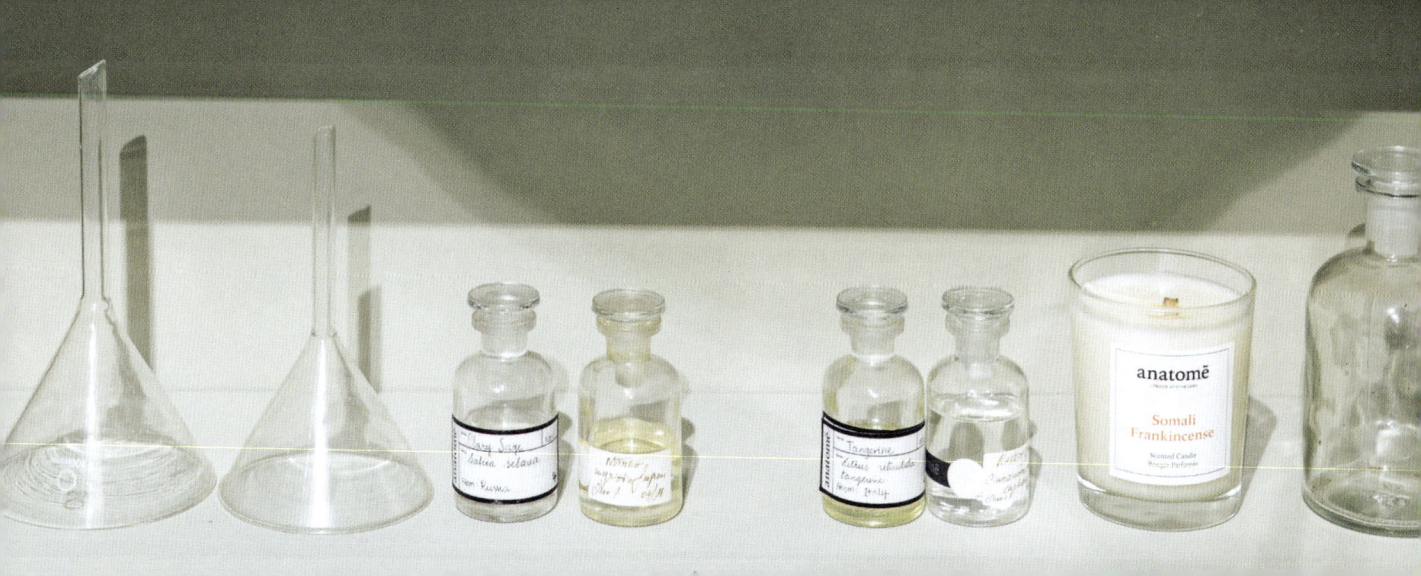

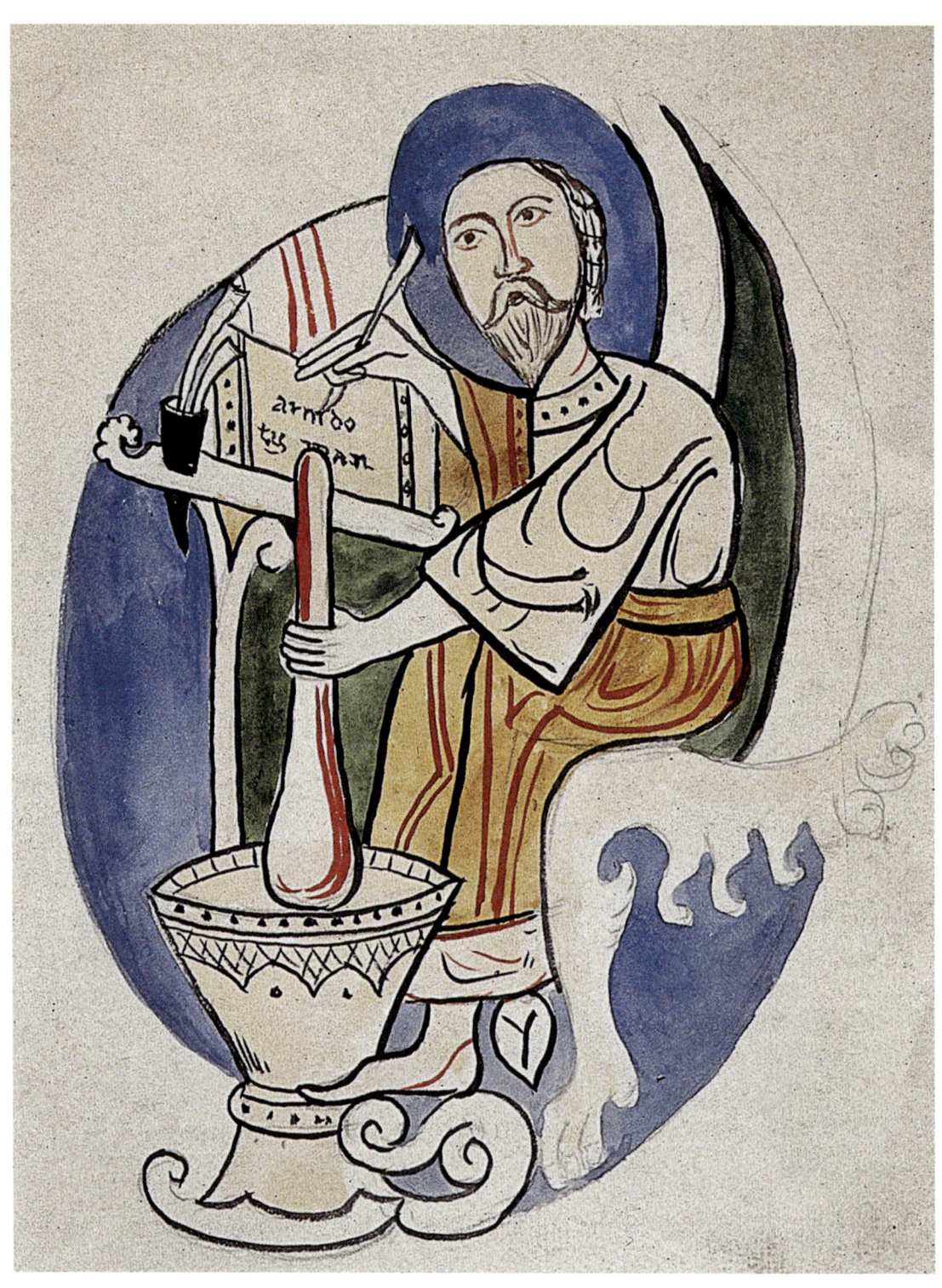

BRANDING WELLBEING THROUGH THE AGES

At given times in history, wellbeing commerçants weren't as clearly defined as they are now. Pharmacists, alchemists, apothecaries and grocers would employ symbols to signify their trade, affirm their authority and appeal to customers – similar to branding practices we find today. Here's an overview of the evolution of signifiers – or logos, to use today's language – within wellbeing.

Pharmacology has been identified by the same signifier since ancient Egyptian times, with records found in an Egyptian papyrus dating from 1550 BC – the oldest piece of medical literature ever discovered. The symbol in question is the mortar and pestle: an insignia that registers with outstanding accuracy and simplicity the tools used to create medicinal preparations for over 6,000 years.

Pharmacy professionals used the equipment of their trade, such as medical substances, mortar and pestles and carboys (pharmaceutical jars), to advertize on shop signs and in trade magazines, while alchemists used hidden symbols to conceal their chemical formulas. Several visual cues are still employed today on medical facilities, drug packaging and pharmacy shelves. We've grown so accustomed to them we forget to ask ourselves what they meant in the first place.

Snakes were present throughout pharmaceutical history, frequently wrapped around a staff. The rod with a snake on it, which the Greek deity of medicine Asclepius carried,

first appeared as a medical emblem in the fifth century BC. Hermes (the Roman deity Mercury), the gods' spokesman, added a second snake to his staff to make the caduceus. The fact that mercury was a significant chemical agent throughout the history of medicine and alchemy may not be a coincidence. A remedy for a snake bite and epilepsy, the central scalp was injected with a mixture of snake venom and evaporated mercury. Hermes and Mercury – the Greek and Roman gods of trade and commerce – make suitable references for the pharmacy trade.

Design is made easier by the caduceus' symmetrical proportions. It was first employed as a printer's mark (colophon) by a book publisher in the fifteenth century. Its connection to medicine was rekindled when a medical publisher adopted it in the early nineteenth century. On nineteenth-century French pharmaceutical labels, snakes were seen wrapped around palm plants. The purpose was to convey a sense of trust, expertise and healing to the consumers.

Another legendary emblem linked to medicine is the Bowl of Hygeia. According to Greek mythology, Hygeia, Asclepius' daughter and attendant, cared for her father's temples while carrying a cup of medicine from which the serpent of knowledge sipped.

The unicorn is another animal symbol frequently used in pharmaceutical branding. The first people to mention it were the ancient Greeks, who saw it as a representation of grace and purity, with a spiralling horn that had the ability to heal, particularly as an antidote to poisons. Narwhal horns were frequently mistaken for the legendary unicorn's horn when they washed up on beaches and, like other animal horns and bones, were ground up for use in medicine. The unicorn is one of the two symbols of the British monarchy – along with the lion – and King James I gave the Society of Apothecaries their charter and coat of arms with the two unicorns in 1617.

From 1908 to 1995, the Wellcome Foundation and Burroughs Wellcome & Co. used the unicorn as their logos. Henry Wellcome's trademark choice was probably motivated by the unicorn horn legend. He clearly stated to the designers that he wanted 'delicacy, and refinement, and grace with vigour and verve' in his unicorn, according to historians Roy Church and E M Tansey.

Although the cause for this relationship is unknown, the crocodile or alligator was connected to alchemy before moving on to pharmacy and chemist stores. It might just have been a means to demonstrate that the chemist had access to the most exotic materials, or it might have been the reptiles' resemblance to another fabled monster, the wyvern, a form of dragon, as suggested by nature writer Hannah Velten. The two-legged wyvern, which signifies sickness, rests atop the god Apollo in the Society of Apothecaries' coat of arms.

In *Romeo and Juliet*, William Shakespeare describes an apothecary in which hangs 'an alligator stuff'd, and other skins of ill-shaped fishes'.

Today, pharmacists mark their locations with a green cross. Early in the twentieth century, the green cross appeared as a medicinal sign for the first time in continental Europe in place of the red cross, which the International Red Cross had adopted in 1863. The Royal Pharmaceutical Society of Great Britain did not adopt the green cross as the official emblem for pharmacies in the country until 1984. The society required that the phrase 'pharmacy' or 'pharmacist' appear with it and that it be produced in a specific shade of green or black and white.

Rx is another another visual representation of the pharmacy industry. It first appeared on prescriptions written by physicians to pharmacists, where it stems from the Roman verb *recipere*, which means 'to take back' or 'to receive'. In America, pharmaceutical products continue to display the symbol, designating a prescription's legitimacy. Though considerably more commonplace than their forerunners, modern pharmaceutical emblems are nonetheless vital as signs of legitimacy and dependability.

THE anatomē SIGNIFIER

During his extensive reading of the history of alchemists, pharmacists, apothecaries and other lesser-known trades linked to wellbeing, anatomē founder Brendan Murdock's head filled with branding ideas for a modern apothecary. It took time – and some distance from tales of the past – to bring anatomē's story to modern days, resignifying wellbeing once again, but keeping a link with the past.

He opted for a stylized, pared-back version of the cross, looking at its graphic weight and rendering it in black over a white background for the ultimate clarity effect. Rather than the pharmaceutical cross, which became synonymous with health and cure, the anatomē logo recalls improvement, bettering and the idea of switching up our wellbeing and adding to our lives.

The result is a perfectly symmetrical 'plus' size with a superscript 'a' on the top left side – a nod to chemical symbols and a subtle recalling of the Rx element used in pharmacies.

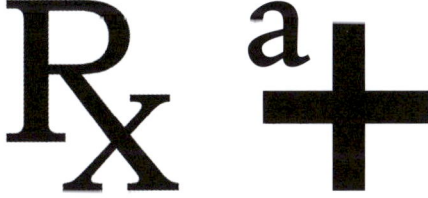

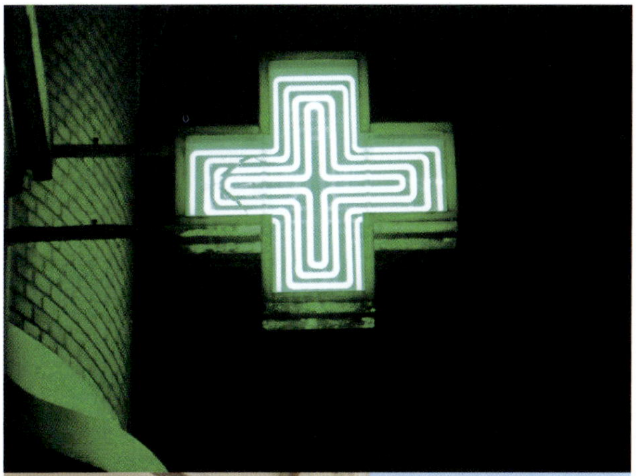

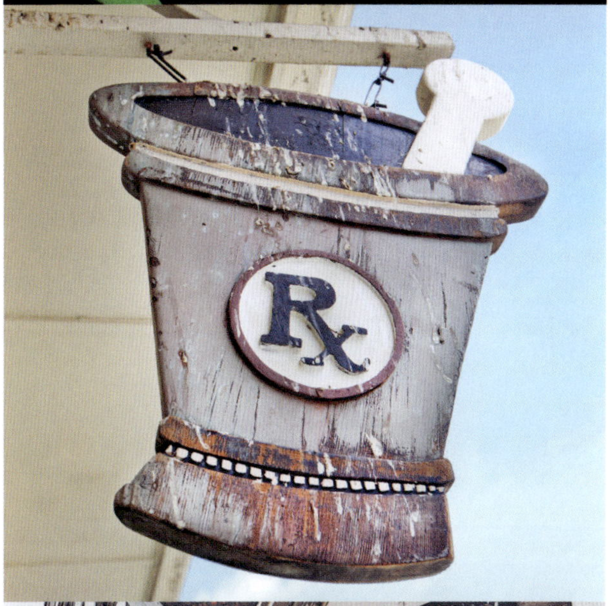

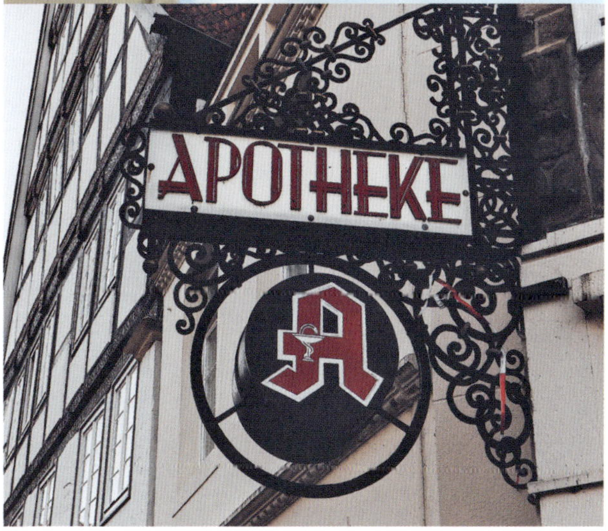

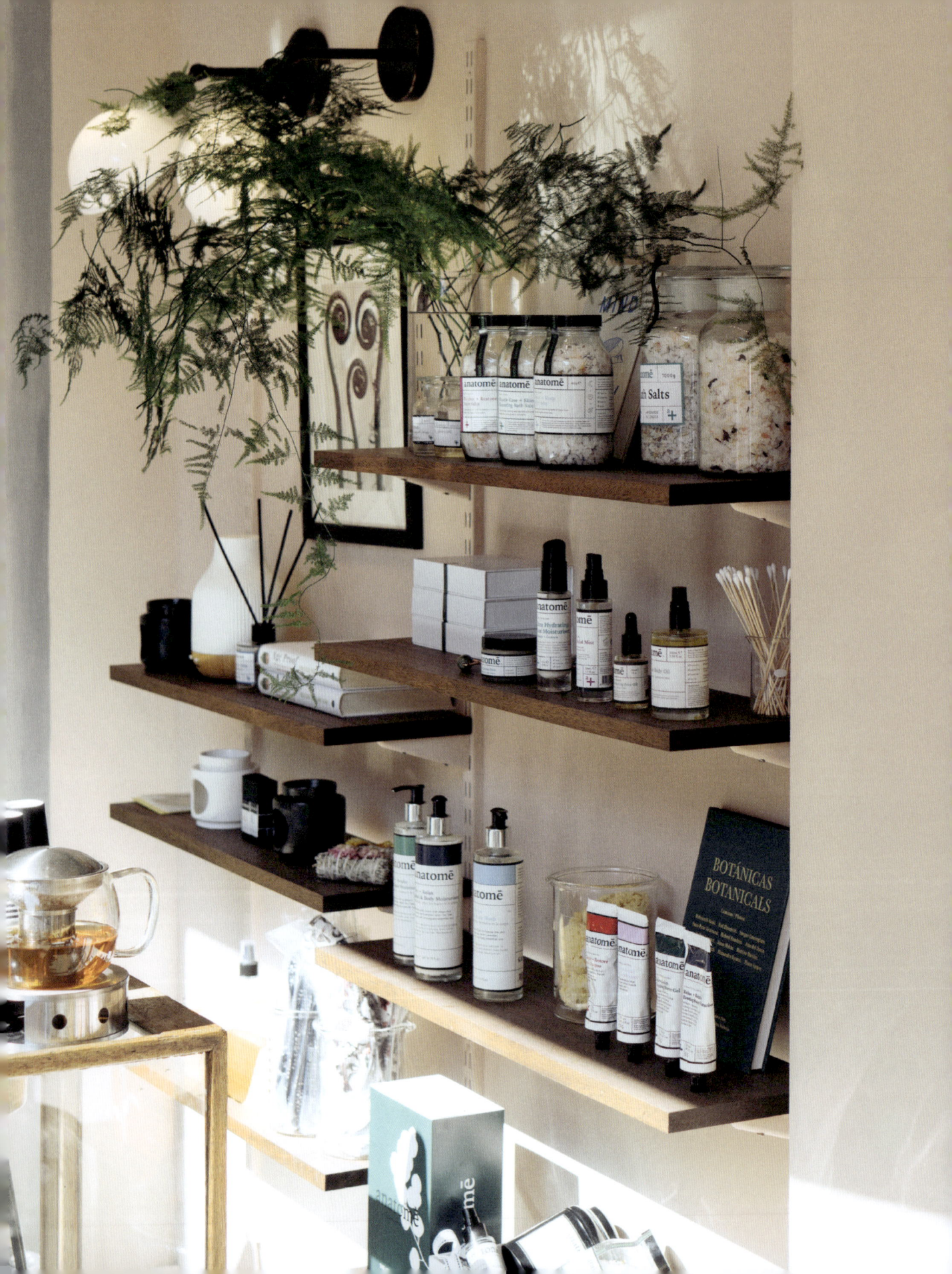

anatomē: LONDON'S MODERN APOTHECARY

anatomē anchors its philosophy in the principles of the apothecaries of the past. Community focus, refined blends and formulations and trust are the pillars of the brand.

The modern apothecary may be inspired by a trade of the past, but it has come a long way from *Sweeney Todd*. Rather than boasting the look and feel of a musty old museum shop, with the help of a team of experts, Brendan Murdock created a fresh, approachable brand ready to help communities feel better: with scents at the centre of it.

The wellbeing offer is infinite, catering to different tastes, lifestyles and yearnings. But it's important to approach wellbeing beyond selling products: anatomē has created – and continues to do so – a lifestyle that puts wellbeing first, making it pleasurable and satisfying.

Not a pharmacy, medical practice, and certainly not a gym, the idea was to provide accessible solutions to wellbeing challenges that come from nature, creating a lifestyle around them and growing a community engaged in feeling better without judgement, pressure or heavy drugs.

Just like apothecaries of the past, Brendan sought to bridge the gap between health and wellness by addressing wellbeing challenges such as sleep, focus, energy, balance and hormonal support: all aspects of everyday life we all feel we can improve but fail to seek information, discuss with others and, finally, tackle.

'Luxury is changing. Instead of accumulating expensive objects, people are discovering the joys of self-care. By offering the best ingredients and helping people take charge of their wellbeing, we're helping them live better. There's nothing more luxurious than that,' Brendan says.

A team of aromachologists, perfumers, and wellbeing specialists support Brendan's creative process. Every new blend and format is carefully studied to contain specific ingredients and feature them in an easy-to-use format, allowing customers to embrace them effortlessly.

Alongside the formulations, community support and lifestyle plans underpin anatomē's activity. Yes, you can buy the product, but adopting self-care practices to make their use more pleasurable and efficient with the support of a dedicated team, will make your wellbeing endeavours more successful.

'Luxury is changing. Instead of accumulating expensive objects, people are discovering the joys of self-care. By offering the best ingredients and helping people take charge of their wellbeing, we're helping them live better. There's nothing more luxurious than that.'

LIFE'S EXLIXIR – THE MUSIC OF DONIZETTI

The idea of anatomē was crystallized after Brendan watched a performance of Gaetano Donizetti's *Elixir of Love* at the Royal Opera House in London. In this nineteenth-century opera, a man, tired of the indifference of his loved woman towards him, seeks a magic potion to help him gain her love.

As the safety curtain came down, it showed old adverts and illustrations of potions and lotions taken from newspapers and magazines of the time. These images triggered a creative wave in Brendan's brain – prompting him to create new, updated versions of potions for the modern consumer.

While Brendan still hasn't yet cracked the recipe to bring love, he had the formulations – and a passion for the history of apothecaries – to bring anatomē to life. All he needed was the codes, language and ideas to update them.

He went back to Shoreditch and, in a warehouse, he set up an apothecary counter. It wasn't about potions – but formulations with scientific backing. And the formulations would help everyone live better. Brendan wanted to help his communities sleep, find focus, perform better and excel at daily activities. That's how they'd find happiness.

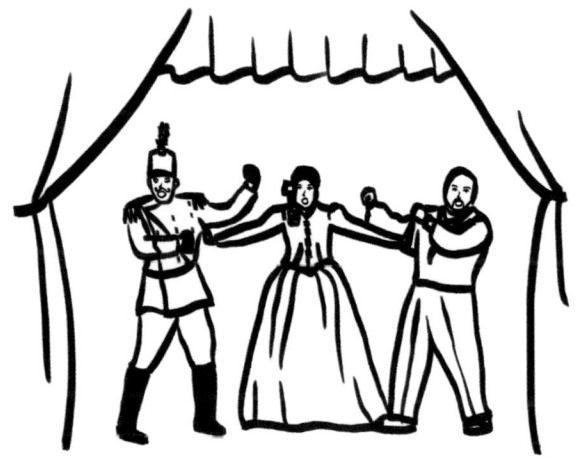

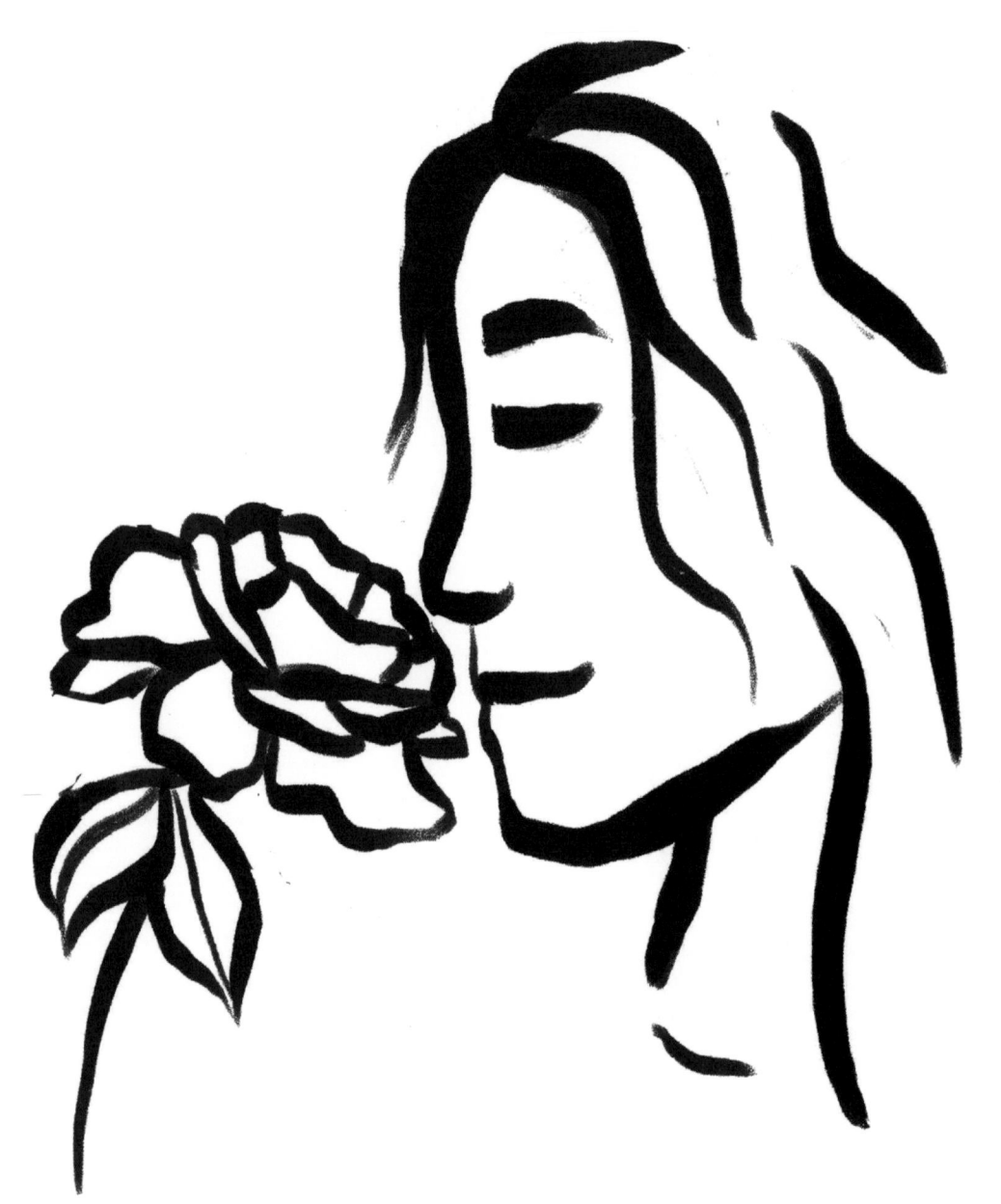

WHAT IS AROMACHOLOGY?

We have talked of apothecary of the past dispensing herbs, spices and remedies. anatomē's approach to the apothecary trade is based on aromachology: the science that studies the influence of odours on human behaviour and examines their co-relation with feelings and emotions. These emotions and feelings include relaxation, exhilaration, libido, sensuality, a sense of happiness, concentration and so on.

Aromas are captured by the nose, travel through our olfactory pathways and end in the brain's limbic system – the part of our brains responsible for behavioural and emotional responses. The study of aromas and their co-relation with psychology is called aromachology.

Scents have a strong connection with feelings and emotions, and can strongly influence human behaviour. An odour – or aroma – can trigger relaxation, exhilaration, libido and sensuality, a sense of happiness, concentration and so on. It's an exciting world where using the power of scent can support your overall wellbeing.

Although studies and observations in this field go back to ancient times, as you will later discover in this book, the term aromachology was created in 1989 by the Sense of Smell Institute (SSI), a division of The Fragrance Foundation. It derives from 'aroma' and 'physio-psychology'.

This science is devoted to identifying and proving the psychological effects of scents, as well as the impact of aromas on the brain, to develop therapies to assess human behaviour and promote mental health benefits, to help you sleep, move and create.

anatomē based its formulations on aromachology findings and medicinal history. Studies have indicated that parts of the brain responsible for alertness and concentration can be influenced by scent.

Throughout this book you will discover how the power of various key botanicals have informed anatomē's oil formulations, all of which have been created for topical use on sensory points to achieve the maximum therapeutic benefits. anatomē's team of aromachologists and nutritionists have carefully developed formulations to bring balance to modern lifestyles by blending ingredients from nature chosen for their positive effect on sleep, diet, skincare and overall health.

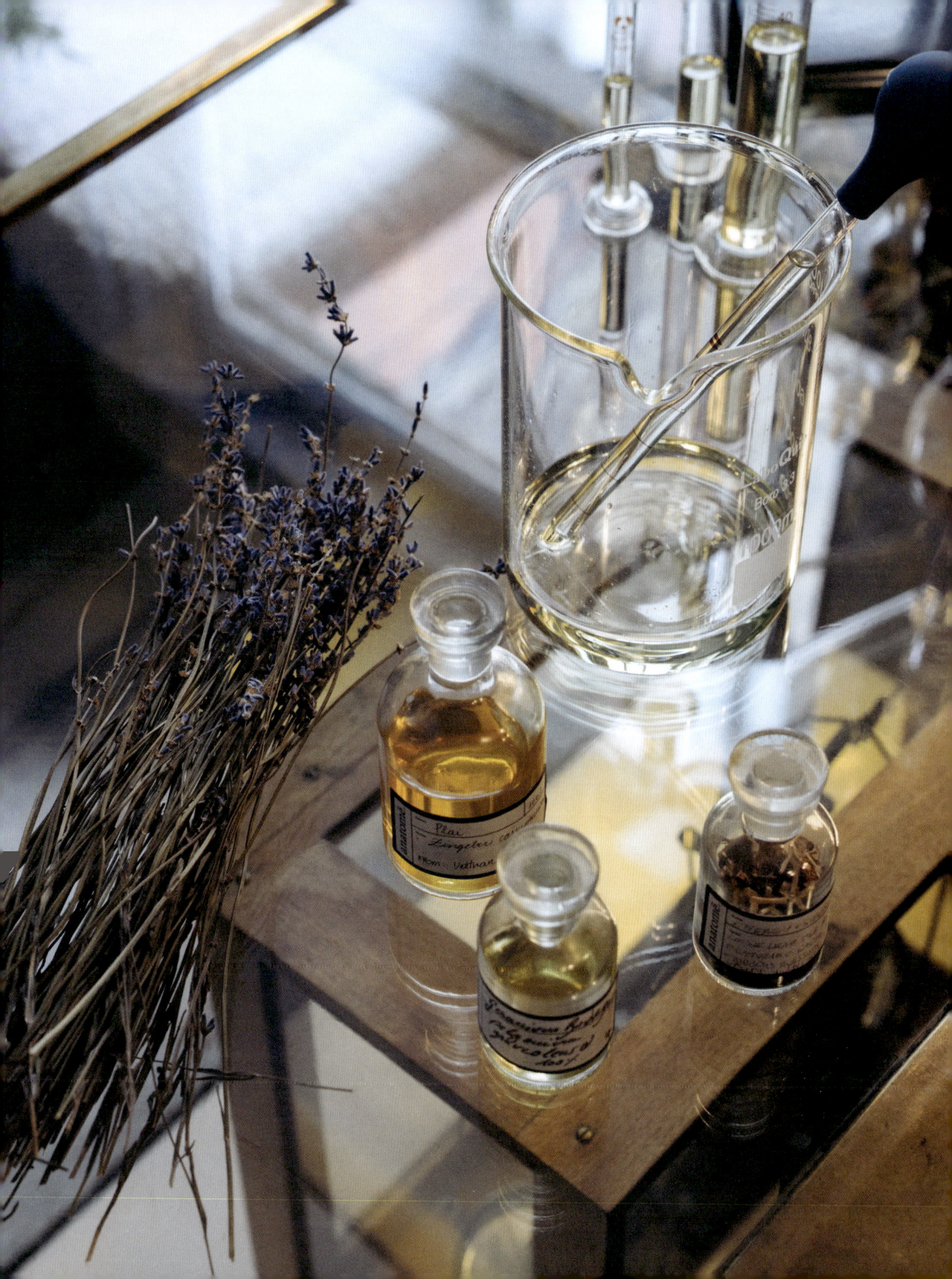

WEL
P

LBEING

ILLARS

TODAY'S WELLBEING YEARNINGS

The term 'wellbeing' refers to the state of being comfortable, healthy and happy. It's a broad term that can refer to mental or physical health. anatomē breaks this down into five pillars of wellbeing: sleep, balance, movement, focus and diet.

Wellbeing is commonly applied to minor health manifestations – feelings and states that we want to improve, but nothing too urgent that requires immediate medical attention.

We can overlook wellbeing aspects, letting them play in the background while we strive to achieve more, earn more, perform, look better or enjoy ourselves.

But an overlooked wellbeing yearning can evolve into more severe physical and mental health conditions. If we find the time to investigate our wellbeing deficits, we can unlock an array of practices that can adjust the cycles, helping us achieve more, feel better and live happier.

Wellbeing is a latent craving for many of us. We want to feel better, but distractions, worries and lifestyle vices keep us from switching our focus toward a better version of ourselves.

We are programmed to function, but not to maintain our 'machinery'. When it comes to our bodies, anatomē believes in cooling engines and keeping machines oiled (pun intended) and allowing time and space for maintenance. Daily. Even if only for a few minutes.

---

anatomē's
WELLBEING ASSESSMENT

On a piece of paper, on your phone, tablet or notebook, answer the following questions:

1 How much of your diet is health-focused?

2 How often do you assess your health from a preventative perspective (check-ups, for instance)?

3 Do you assess minor, ongoing health challenges or carry on life with them playing in the background?

4 How much time daily do you dedicate to feeling good (including exercise, meditation, downtime and rest)?

5 How much sleep do you get daily?

If your answers have revealed a hedonistic personality with little downtime; a workaholic with reckless health behaviour; or an altruistic family person who never puts yourself first, don't worry: **you're perfectly normal.**

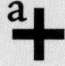

1
SLEEP

Human beings spend 25–35 per cent of their lives sleeping. Until the mid-twentieth century, we believed sleep was the body's dormant state when we switched ourselves off to passively 'recover'. Studies then began to show a completely different reality. As it turns out, sleeping is a busy time for our brains when they perform a series of vital activities. These functions are directly related to how we spend 75–65 per cent of our lives.

This understanding helped build anatomē. We believe that ingredients that support better sleep, aligned with a series of practices and habits, help us kickstart a journey towards better mental and physical health.

As such, this book contains at least 35 per cent sleep-related information – mirroring real life. We recommend you don't sleep through this part. It's all valuable information and, once digested, should help you sleep through to enjoy a better time awake.

We've come a long way in our perception of sleep and its importance to our bodies, particularly throughout the twentieth century – the research during this period has shifted our approach to the subject.

SLEEP AND THE IMMUNE SYSTEM

Science has shown us that lack of sleep is directly linked to immunity deficiency. When we don't sleep enough, we become more vulnerable to infections and take longer to recover from diseases. Here's how:

Cytokines are proteins released by our immune system. They help promote sleep, and also to protect us from infections and inflammations, and even help control our stress.

That is why, when we're unwell, we tend to feel tired and sleepier: we need more cytokines. Less sleep, fewer cytokines. Fewer cytokines, less protection.

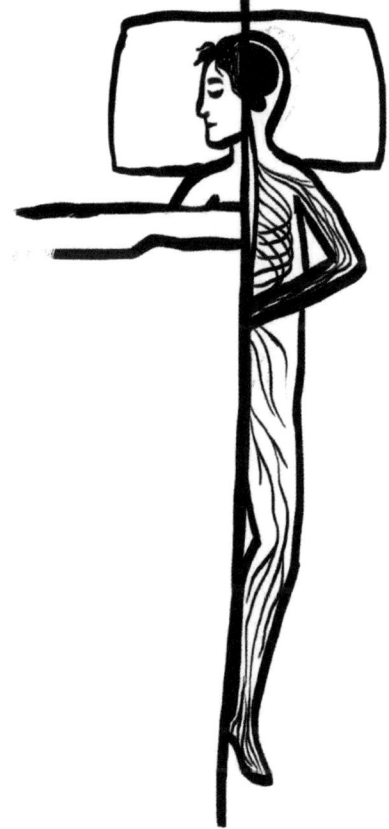

SLEEP, HORMONES AND THE NERVOUS SYSTEM

The chemicals in our brains responsible for sleep are called neurotransmitters. They control the communications of our nerves, telling the rest of the body what to do. Neurotransmitters called serotonin and noradrenaline, which keep our bodies awake, are produced by neurons in the brainstem, where the brain and the spinal cord connect. When we're asleep, the work happens in the base of the brain, where neurons turn off the awakeness signs.

Our sympathetic nervous system – in charge of controlling fight, flight or freeze responses – relaxes while we sleep. This fundamental function controls our blood pressure. Studies have proven that sleep-deprived individuals are more likely to develop coronary disease due to high blood pressure.

During our non-rapid eye movement sleep cycles (NREM), we may experience vivid dreams. During this cycle, our muscles cannot move – a fascinating bodily function, allowing us to live our dreams without physically reacting to them (and potentially hurting or scaring someone sleeping next to us).

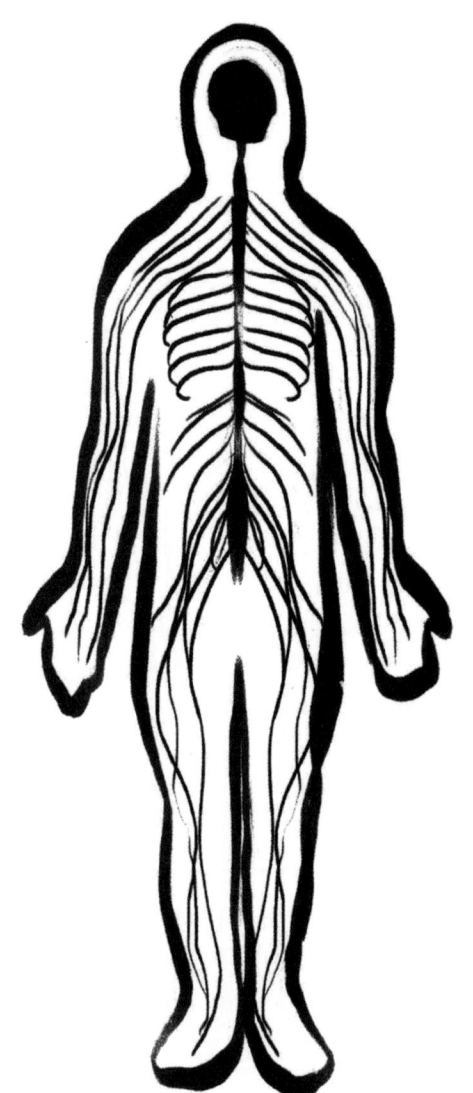

You've probably heard that sleep is a vital part of any weight-loss programme. Here's the scientific reason: during our early sleep, our levels of the stress hormone, cortisol, decrease before going up again as wake-up time approaches, giving us that perky feel and switching our appetite on.

Amongst the many hormones our bodies release during sleep, melatonin is in charge of our sleep patterns. Its levels increase at night, giving us a sleepy feeling and telling our bodies it's time to hit the bed.

Also during our sleep, the pituitary gland releases growth hormone, responsible for body growth in children and repair in adults.

SLEEP AND ESSENTIAL OILS

The use of aromatic compounds for promoting sleep has been rooted in traditional medicine systems in practice for centuries. Research on the subject had significant studies emerging in the 1990s and early 2000s, providing an evidence-based understanding of their benefits.

Inhalation of specific essential oils stimulates olfactory receptors, which send signals to the limbic system, the brain's emotional centre. This interaction activates neurotransmitters like serotonin and gamma-aminobutyric acid (GABA), which promote relaxation and reduce anxiety.

anatomē's sleep formulations are created to harvest the benefits of key ingredients, each tackling a specific sleep pattern. We use Himalayan and Cornish Lavender oil to support the stressed mind: it contains linalool, a compound with sedative properties that can increase slow-wave sleep and decrease heart rate (for more on the power of lavender, see page 172). Roman Chamomile oil possesses anxiolytic properties, making it most suited for restless sleepers. Meanwhile, Somali Frankincense oil has shown the potential to reduce cortisol levels, the primary stress hormone, promoting relaxation, alleviating anxiety and supporting overactive minds.

SLEEP AND RECENT MEMORY

Before an exam, a work presentation or an interview, we spend the remaining hours preceding the crucial intellectual task preparing for it. We may have little to no sleep, focusing on the big event and reviewing every piece of information we need to remember the following day.

We finally feel we've either done all the work we can – or enough to get through – and go to bed. Rather than the 6–8 hours of needed sleep, we get only 2–3 hours.

The moment comes. Suddenly, the precious information we had spent time and energy storing in our brains seems to disappear. And it was gone as if it'd never been there.

We blame it on fatigue. Nerves. We blame it on the examiner or interviewer. And, while they all may play their part, chances are we've forgotten to give our brains the time needed to process the information – an activity it performs while we are asleep.

While studies on the matter are relatively recent and ongoing, we've learned much about sleep and our ability to store information:

- While we sleep, newly acquired memory is protected from disruptions from events that may happen during wakefulness.
- During sleep, our brains classify the information recently acquired by likely importance, as well as our remembering needs.

As such, while we kept ourselves awake to prepare, we didn't classify, didn't store or make the information correctly available in our brains, so when the time comes to retrieve the information, it's not where we wanted or expected it to be. It's as if we'd dropped a book on the floor of a large library while walking around and returned the following day trying to find the same dropped book on its correct shelf.

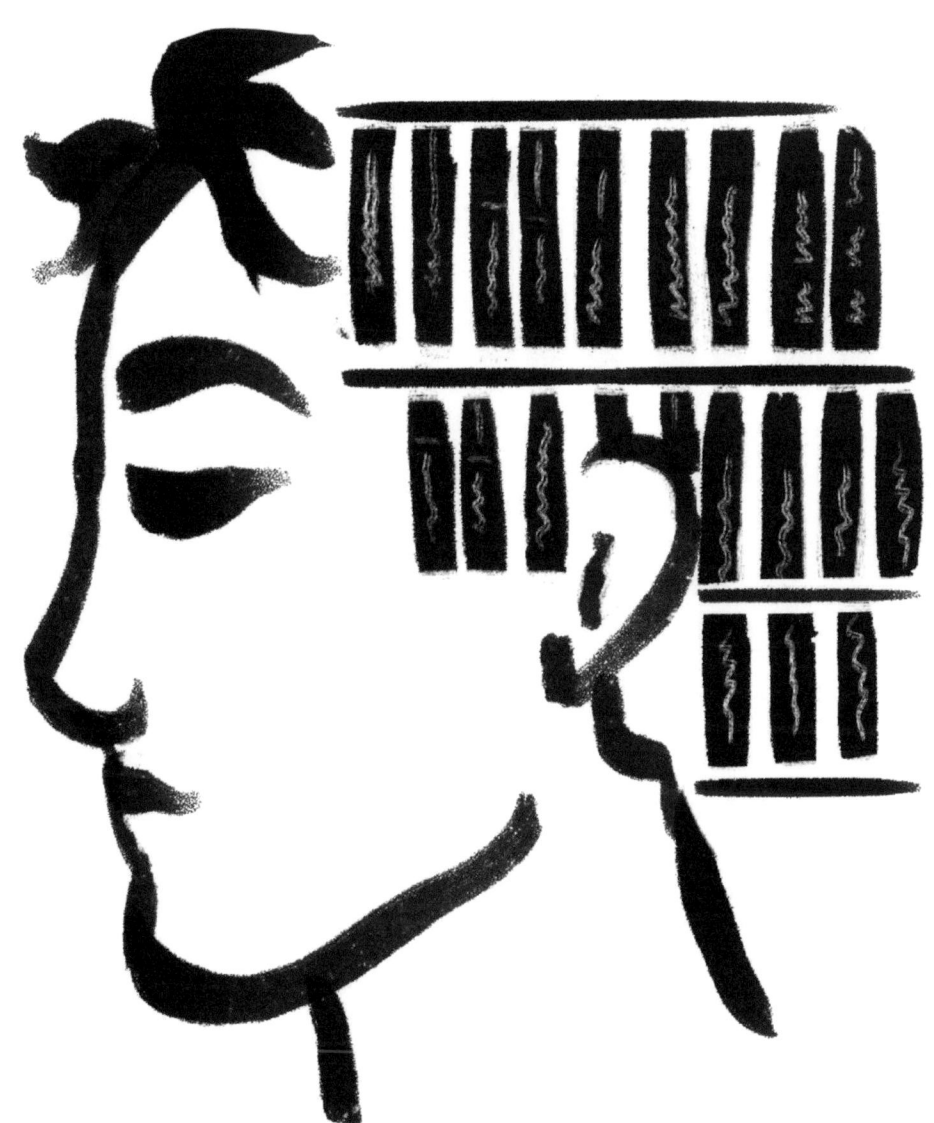

WELLBEING PILLARS

53

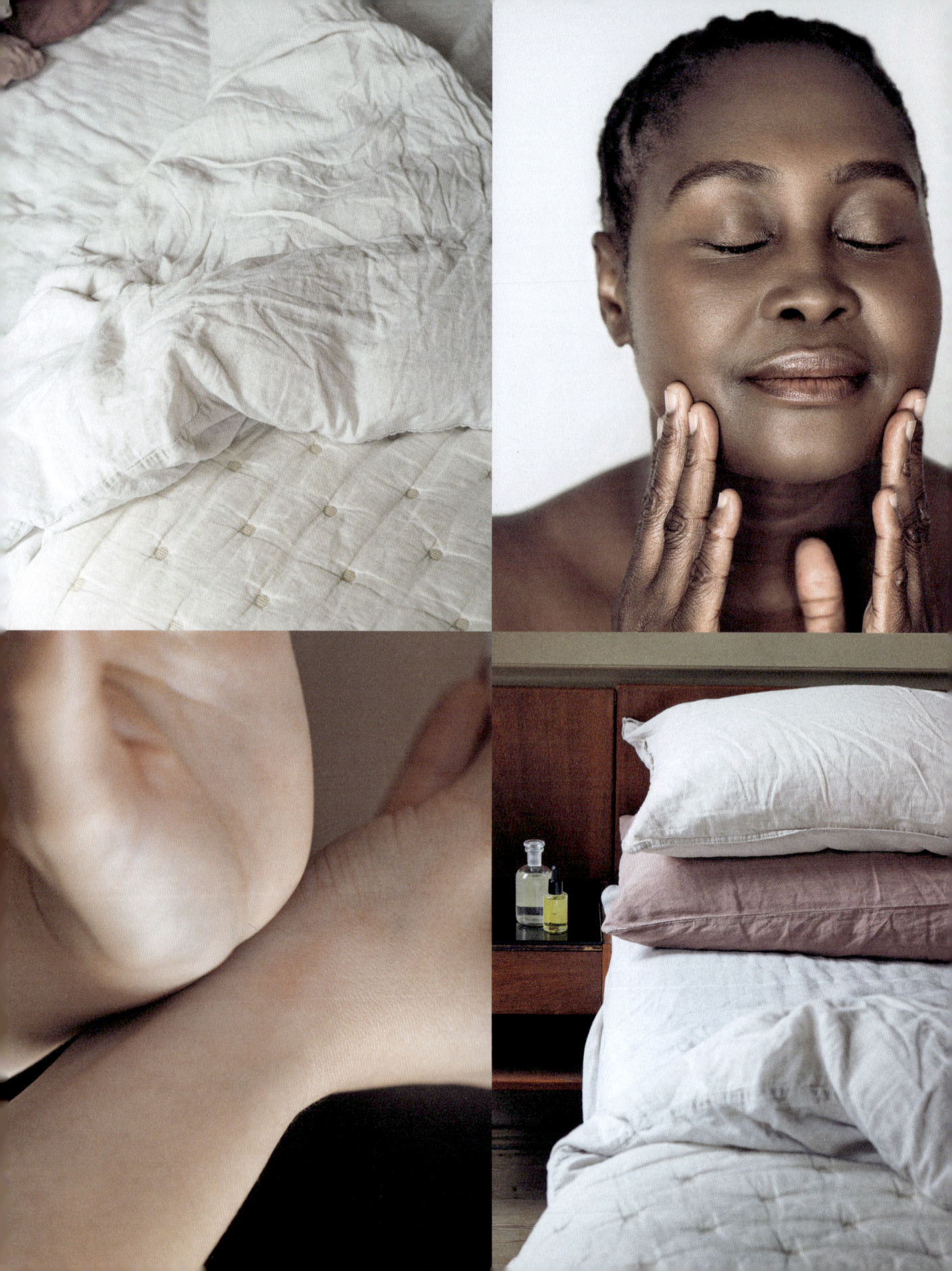

SLEEP AND BEAUTY

Here are a few things you may not know about 'beauty sleep'. Keep reading: it can help turn back the clock on your appearance.

COLLAGEN

Collagen is a structural protein in the body's connective tissues, including joints and deeper layers of our skin, giving it sustenance, volume and a healthy appearance. The production of this protein reduces with age, leading to joint pain and sagging, wrinkly skin.

Collagen synthesis happens during our sleep as a part of our repair process. When you sleep only for only 5 hours or less, collagen production is affected, making your skin look saggy. Switch back to 8 hours, and you'll swiftly regain plumpness and smoothness. Keep sleep consistent, and your collagen production will be high and paced, slowing down the ageing process and the appearance of new lines and wrinkles.

THAT HEALTHY GLOW

We all love the look of a morning after a good night's sleep (once the puffiness gets washed away with cold water). We can explain this rested look. During our sleep, our bodies pump more blood to our skin vessels. This extra blood flow gives us rosier cheeks, replenishes skin cells and results in glowing, youthful-looking skin. That's why we suggest using a face treatment with avocado oil at night to help give the skin extra nourishment when you sleep.

WE CAN SEE IT IN YOUR EYES

Wearing sunglasses in the office after a big night out to hide the redness and the dark circles: does it ring a bell? While this dreadful look is a result of too little sleep and the potential effects of alcohol, a daily sleep deficit may be the cause of your continuous dreaded dark circles and lifeless eyes. Before you resort to needles, try a combination of hydration, a slightly elevated pillow and 8 hours of rest. Add a hydrating balm or serum for the eyes in the morning, and you'll be in control of your tired look.

SLEEP POSITIONS: IS THERE A CORRECT ONE?

At the first sign of pain and stiffness, unless we know for sure what caused it, we revisit our sleep position (or someone does it for us). Everyone has an opinion – or something they heard – to share. And they're often confusing.

The first aspect to consider when assessing your sleep position is your spine alignment. However you choose to sleep, you must maintain your vertebrae in a straight row and supported, allowing blood circulation, relieving pressure on spinal tissues and promoting muscle relaxation and recovery.

Sleep positions vary from one individual to another. Factors such as body shape, weight, pregnancy, acid reflux and other health conditions will influence the assessment.

The best positions for a healthy spine are either on your side or your back. That is due to the direct mattress support and the reduced pressure on organs, compared with sleeping on your front.

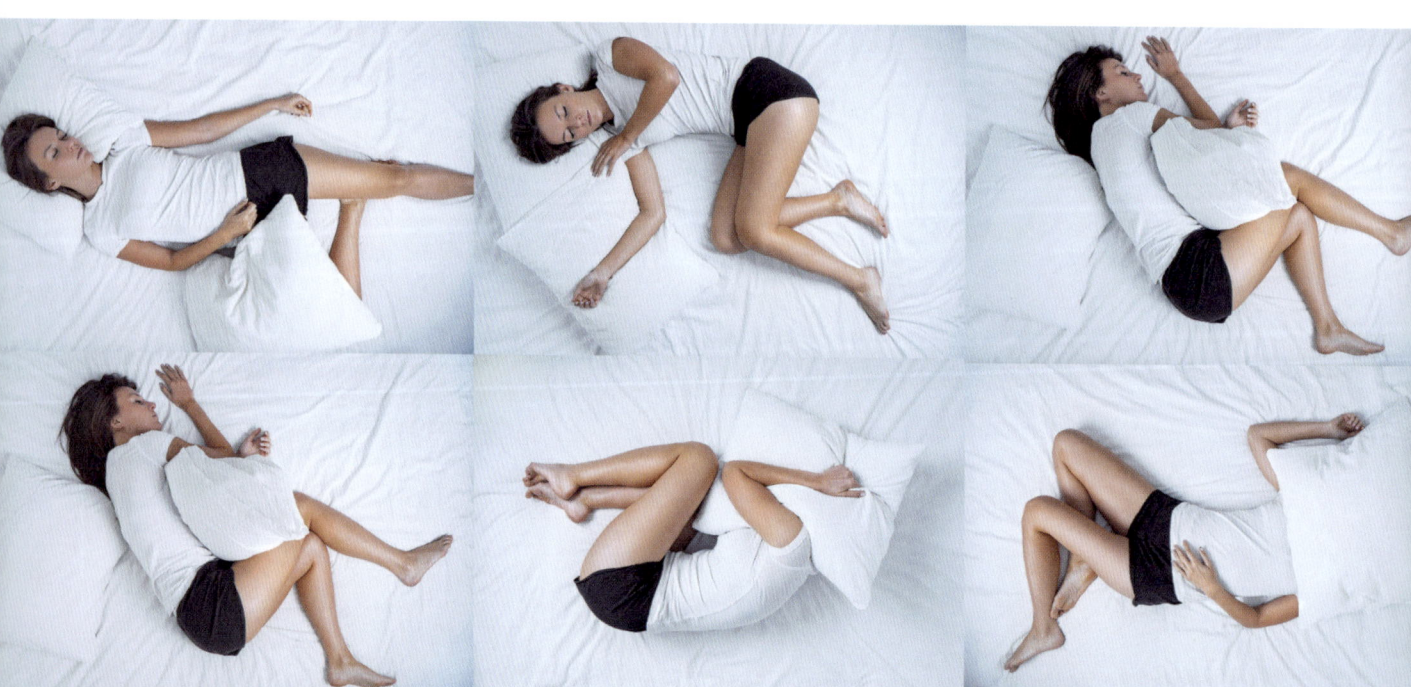

SLEEPING ON YOUR SIDE

About 60 per cent of adults sleep on their side, as it's more comfortable. It promotes spine alignment and, with the support of pillows, is considered the safest position to avoid back pain. Sleeping on your side is also the best way to reduce heartburn, particularly when combined with an elevated neck and head (always consider your spine alignment when embracing this sleep position).

SLEEPING ON YOUR BACK

The second favourite position, sleeping on the back, comes with a list of benefits. And they're different from side sleep. Efficient in promoting spine alignment, it helps distribute body weight evenly, preventing back or neck pains, and keeps limbs free from pressure, preventing aches, pinched nerves and numbness. This position also has beauty benefits. When your face is upward, it isn't pressing against pillows or mattresses, which helps avoid creases and wrinkles.

SLEEPING ON YOUR STOMACH

The least popular, accounting for 10 per cent of people. Supporting the ribs to avoid pressure on the chest means muscle strain, which can promote less restful sleep. That said, sleeping on your stomach can be the best choice to relieve snoring by opening the airways.

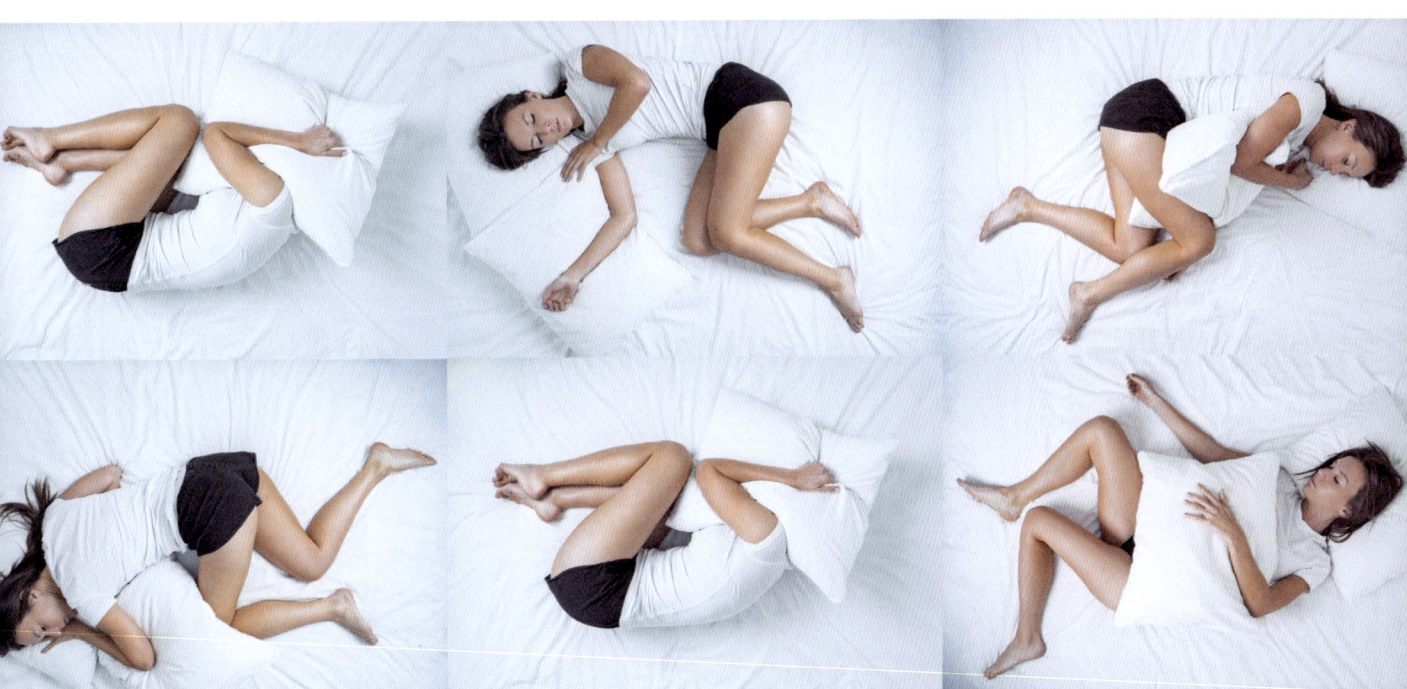

SLEEP THROUGH THE AGES

While humans have always slept, the concept of sleep hasn't always been seen in the same way by different civilisations over time. Sleep has been described in various ways by ancient Indian sages, Egyptians, Greeks and Romans, with many of these ancient societies assigning specific deities to dreams, and interpreting dream themes in different ways.

Around 450 BC

Greek physician Alcmaeon believed that sleep was a period of unawareness caused by diminished blood circulation in the brain as a result of blood exiting the body's outer layer.

162 AD

Galen suggested that the brain, rather than the heart, was responsible for consciousness.

Throughout the following centuries, not much was achieved in terms of grasping the concept of sleep. Indeed, it was perceived as a detoxifying procedure, one that put certain bodily functions to sleep, or attributes its onset to a lack of blood flow.

In the Age of Enlightenment, some scientific experts began studying their dreams as a practice. The bedroom shifted to become a place for sleep and sexual intimacy only. During this time, physicians began to determine how much one should sleep.

It was only in the 1800s that getting too much rest began to be seen as a sign of idleness.

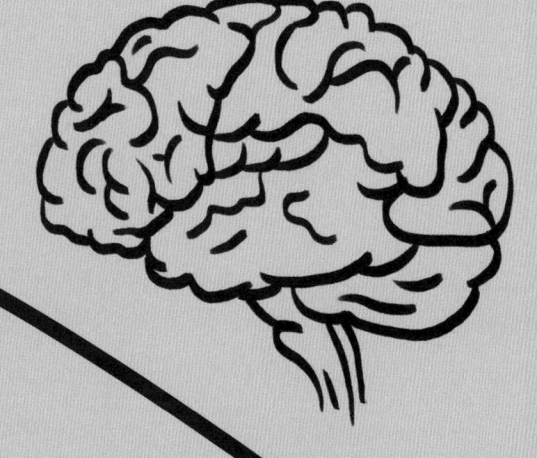

Around 400 BC

People believed that the decrease in temperature of someone asleep was responsible for making them drowsy.

Aristotle speculated that sleep was a suspension of consciousness in the heart, believed to be the source of both feeling and reason. He also connected digestive activity with the beginning of sleep.

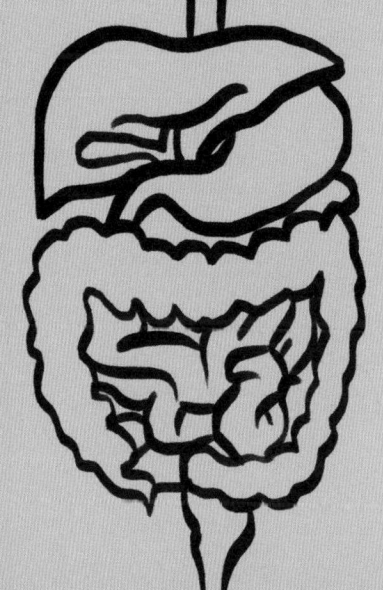

1900s

Neurons were considered the individual units of the nervous system, a discovery followed by the formulation of the first ever sleeping pill: barbital. This invention changed societal behaviour, quickly becoming one of the most misused substances in the United States within 30 years.

Another breakthrough during this time was the discovery of circadian rhythms: the natural, internal 24-hour biological cycles that regulate various physiological and behavioural processes in living organisms.

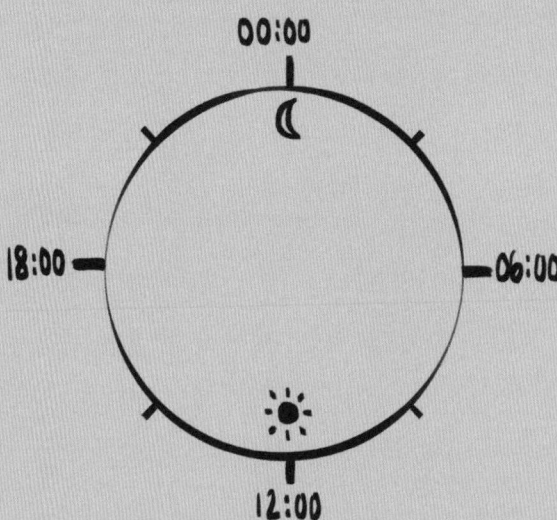

1920s

Nathaniel Kleitman became a distinguished scientist in the realm of sleep pathophysiology. By 1925, he had made his first groundbreaking discovery: rapid eye movement (REM) sleep. His research expanded to include other aspects of sleep and wakefulness, such as mental activity, consciousness, voluntary movement and the ramifications of sleep deprivation.

In 1924 The electroencephalogram (EEG) was developed, unveiling the varying electrical brain waves in wakefulness and sleep. At roughly the same time, stimulants started to be used to keep narcolepsy patients awake.

1910s

Henri Piéron discovered that sleep-deprived animals secreted a sleep-inducing molecule into the cerebrospinal fluid. He named it 'hypnotoxin'. This molecule could make alert dogs fall into a deep sleep when injected into them. Two years later, Piéron published the first book to attempt to discuss sleep physiology called *Le problème physiologique du Sommeil* in 1913.

Constantin von Economo, a pyschiatrist and neurologist, researched encephalitis patients with irregular sleep patterns in1916. As a result of his work, he found the hypothalamus in the brain was responsible for both sleeping and wakefulness.

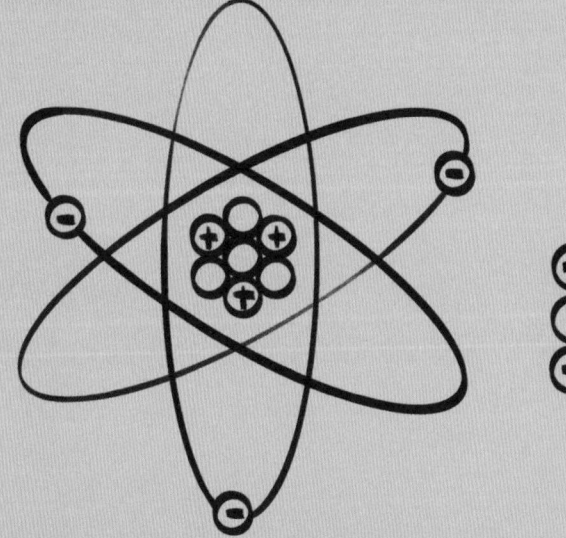

1960s

In 1962, pioneering researcher Michel Jouvet discovered that a structure within the brainstem called the pons regulated REM sleep.

Obstructive sleep apnea made its mark on sleep medicine in 1965 as scientists studied the physiological changes associated with slumber and awakening. This study was reinforced by a detailed scrutiny of temperature, blood flow and breathing while asleep.

Dr Roger Broughton established that bed-wetting and disruptive sleep-related discorders (parasomnias) were caused by a disordered transition out of slow-wave sleep rather than REM in 1968.

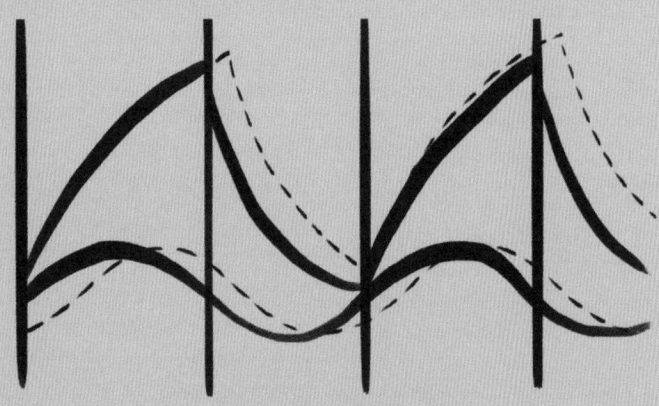

1970–1990

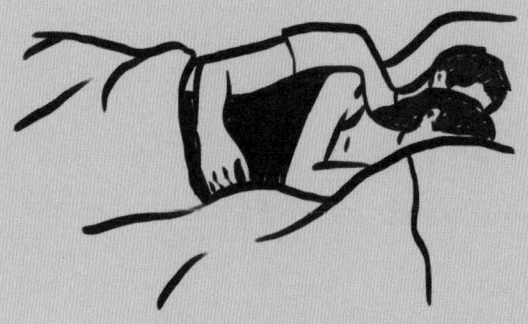

The first specialized sleep research centre is installed at Stanford. In addition, researchers identified a gene ('per') plus a physical location (suprachiasmatic nucleus) for circadian rhythms and developed reliable methods for measuring drowsiness, such as the multiple sleep latency test (MSLT).

Further connections between circadian rhythms and how long we sleep are discovered, in addition to other stimuli. Scientists began to explore the relationship between sleeping and learning and its necessity for survival. Molecular biology began to make a significant impact, leading to the publication of *Principles and Practice of Sleep Medicine* in 1989 – an influential work on sleep studies.

2
BALANCE

External and internal factors affect our mood daily. While
the challenges of mental health increase, and awareness,
open discussions and support should be at the top of our
minds, we often neglect minor, often frequent, signs of
mood imbalance.

It all varies from one individual to another. And it often requires someone else
to point out when we're 'in a bad mood'. While an angry email, a muffled insult
to a stranger or even a short fuse at home are part of modern life, controlling and
reducing the occurrence of these episodes, avoiding a spiralling of negativity, can
be one of the most beneficial actions for your wellbeing.

Balance practices are well known. We know how a spa day can switch up our
mood, or purchasing a new bag can temporarily numb the effects of a difficult
week at work. But, more sustainably, what can we do to restore ourselves?

We believe in a daily mood check and a little dusting of our angry selves to
restore a sense of balance. Here's the anatomē guide to restoring a serene sense
of self.

IDENTIFY THE ORIGIN OF YOUR MOOD IMBALANCE

Easier said than done, we know. But you may be able to identify patterns in your lifestyle that trigger your behaviour. We will list some of the most common sources of 'bad mood', and will leave you to, without self-judgement, come to conclusions. Then we will offer comprehensive support and ideas that won't drastically change your routine. Stick with us.

- **Alcohol**, despite its delightful effect of momentary numbing, its convivial fabulousness and all the pleasures we know so well, can – and does – affect your levels of serotonin and dopamine: the chemicals in your brain in charge of keeping you happy. Can you identify a grumpier mood the day after you consume more alcohol? Even a slight increase in alcohol intake can trigger anxiety or feelings of depression.

- **Diet** is another crucial factor in the maintenance of your mood. Excessive sugar and refined carbohydrates may trigger fluctuations in the glucose levels in your blood, causing irritation and lack of energy. Skipping meals or having inconsistent nutritional schedules will also trigger the same issues.

- **Environmental factors**, although subjective and broad, are also to blame for a decrease in good-mood levels. If you can identify a life pattern, a relationship or a habit that makes you unhappy, do not ignore it. There are ways of shifting your mindset to manage unavoidable environmental factors and create mechanisms that make you more resistant to mood-harming situations.

HOW TO BECOME MORE BALANCED

CONTROL STRESS

- **It's pointless to tell someone 'not to stress'.** Stress is a part of being alive in the twenty-first century. It can originate from internal issues, external issues that we can control, external issues out of our control and macro events (such as war, climate change or political and societal challenges).

- **We won't advise you on how to eradicate stress** or manage its sources, as they're too varied for anatomē to tackle. We can, however, help you prioritize, mute unneeded information and find escapism and relativisation to reduce the impact of stress in your life.

- **If your stress is functional** – related to your daily activities – investing in your time management skills will help ease the impact of busyness on your life. It can be as simple as writing a priority-ordered to-do list.

- **If your stress is emotional**, managing it is a matter of relativization and lifestyle hygiene. If you're suffering from deeper or clinical mental health issues such as depression and anxiety, your first step is to assess them with the help of a professional. If the source is simply an accumulation of everyday feelings that you believe you can manage, a 360-degree wellbeing assessment will help diminish the impact of your thoughts.

- **Breathing exercises** can be beneficial if you experience anxiety, general stress and restlessness. Taking 10 minutes of your day to breathe mindfully will help you be present and diminish your stress. We have a breathing guide on page 141 to help get you started.

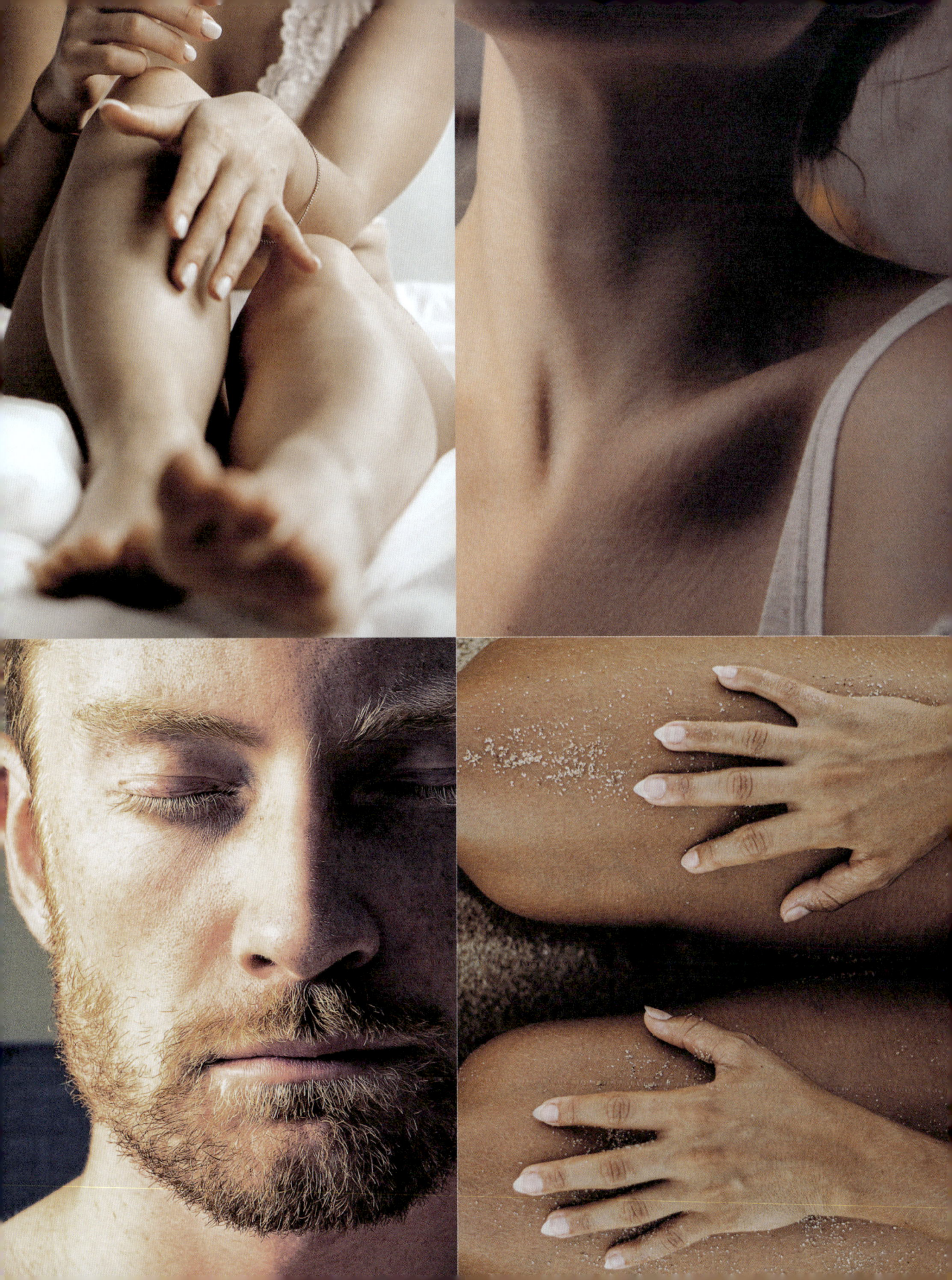

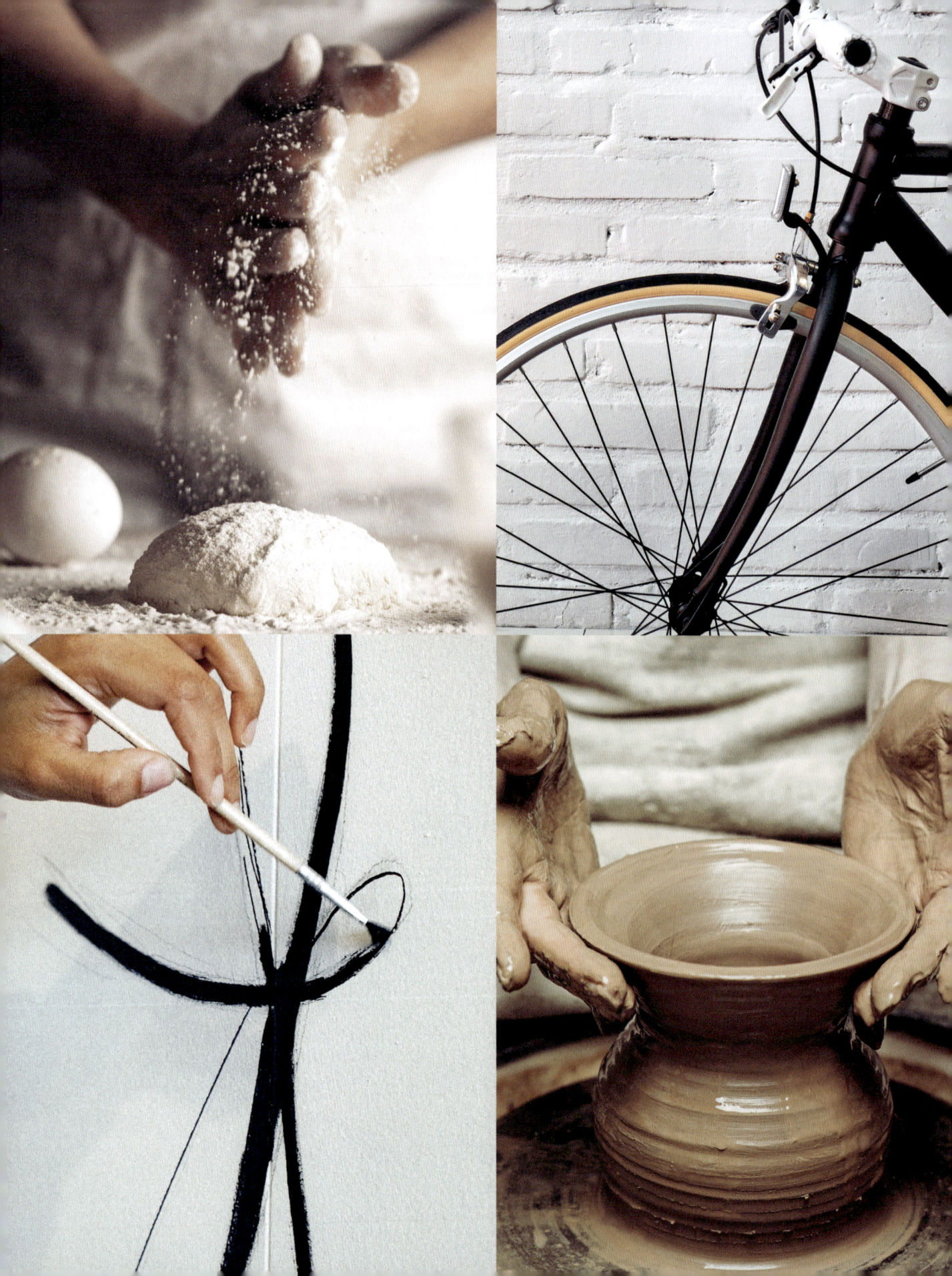

DO MORE OF WHAT YOU LOVE

Before you skim through this part and go on a drinking binge, shopping spree or fast-food fest, let's filter the pleasurable activities in your life, separating 'sheer indulgence' to 'life-enhancing feel-good moments'.

Forget the quick fixes that generate post-enjoyment guilt – and increase stress. Anything involving a negative aftermath should trigger an internal alarm to keep your choices in check. You want to focus on enjoyable activities that build a positive aftermath – choices that keep on giving.

According to research, people with hobbies are less likely to experience stress, depressive symptoms and bad mood. You may feel happier and more at ease after engaging in activities that get you moving around or prefer to spend time alone. But having an activity that serves as an antidote to your low mood, and dedicating time to it, will pay off.

A good example is indulging a side of you understimulated in your everyday life. For example, if you work with numbers and spreadsheets but have a penchant for drawing, carving as little as a weekly hour to develop a drawing journal will help switch up your balance.

If you stop scrolling when you see a cooking reel, why not save it, get the ingredients and make time to try the recipe? (It doesn't matter if you don't succeed, by the way.) The options are endless and varied.

You may not even know what floats your boat and increases your happiness. If that's the case, start with a soul-searching exercise. Make sure it's within your budget, healthy, sustainable and not imposed, but 100 per cent your choice.

MIND HORMONAL IMBALANCES

Hormones significantly impact our brain chemistry, affecting our mental health whenever there's an imbalance. Although in different ways, men and women can both suffer from hormonal fluctuations affecting their moods.

Women's emotions are influenced by oestrogen, progesterone and testosterone, particularly during pregnancy, menopause or due to other health conditions. Meanwhile, men will suffer from low moods whenever their testosterone is low.

These hormonal imbalances often come with accompanying symptoms, constituting more complex scenarios. If after a health assessment you detect an imbalance, treat your condition with the help of a doctor, but don't forget the other practices to boost your journey towards a better mood (see pages 64–67).

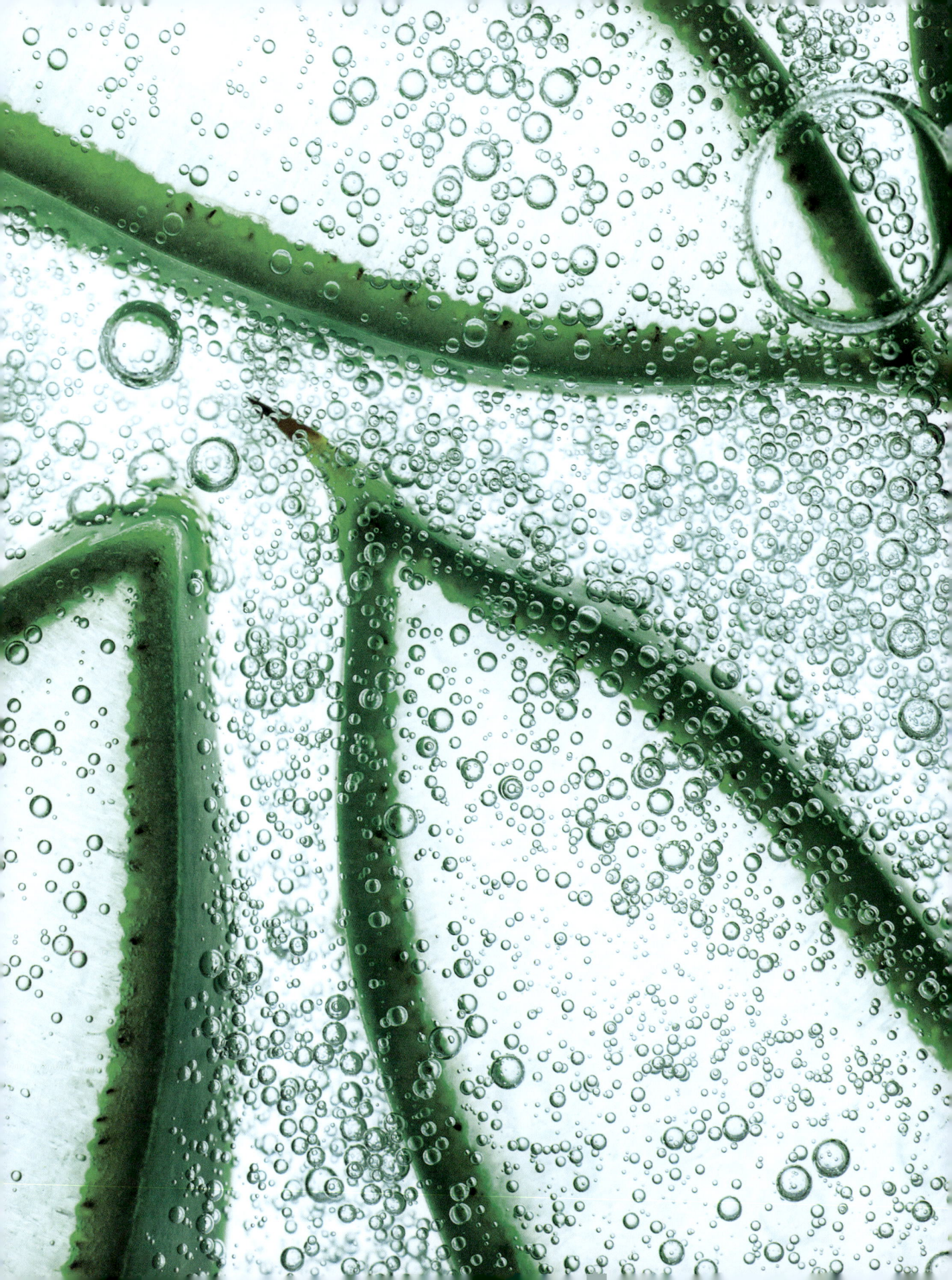

3

MOVEMENT

Movement comprises all activities in which our skeletal muscles make our bodies move, using energy. Exercise is an intensified, dedicated form of movement concentrated in a period. We will discuss the concept of movement comprehensively: we want to promote better health and wellbeing without burdening or asking for drastic changes.

Physically active people live better. They find it easier to control their weight, have a far lower risk of developing heart disease, hypertension, strokes, diabetes and even cancers, and generally have better mental health.

A recent study revealed that 25 per cent of adults are sedentary – or spend more than the recommended waking hours physically inactive. While we like study-backed numbers when it comes to formulating our advice and creating practices, the conversations with our community reveal even more interesting facts and, in this case, numbers.

In consultations, workshops, online questions and in-store conversations, a staggeringly high (we don't keep an exact count) number of our customers revealed not being satisfied with their physical activity amounts. It's a concern amongst those seeking better sleep, trying to find balance and going through life changes.

Even people who exercise regularly have expressed dissatisfaction with their movement routines, often blaming their busy lives for not being able to make enough time to look after their physical health. Others mentioned a lack of motivation and interest, responding to the questions with closed answers such as 'I hate the gym' or 'I don't have discipline'.

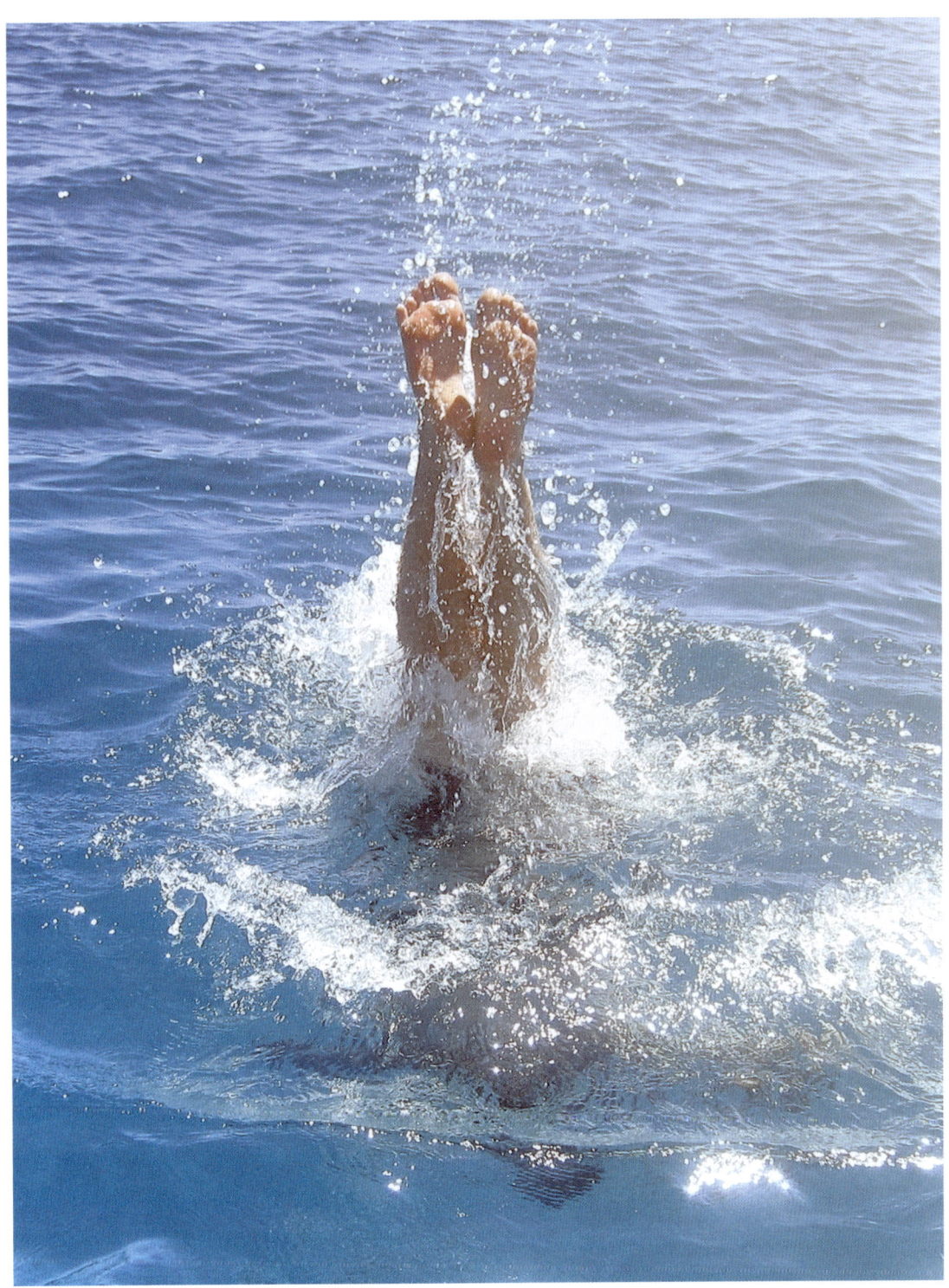

WELLBEING PILLARS

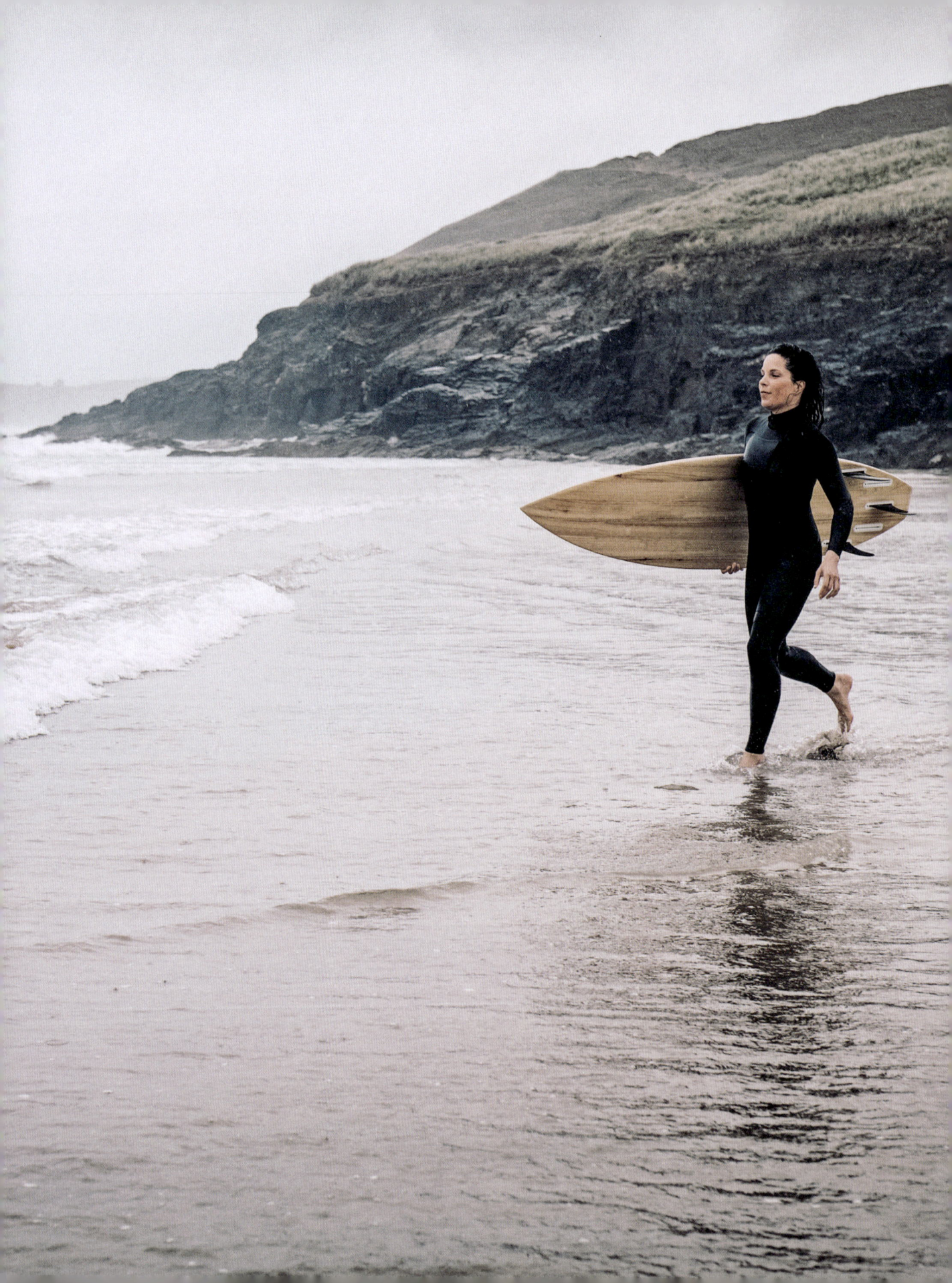

Finally, with a chicken-or-egg situation, many of us get caught in the sedentarism vicious circle, unable to move more and better, suffering from lack of movement, and adding guilt to the picture. Without repeating what you've likely already learned about the benefits of exercise, we take a dynamic approach to movement with encouraging maths we worked out at anatomē. We will show you a few tangential exits from this sendentary circle to increase your daily physical activity.

GET YOUR ENDORPHINS WORKING

The fit people you cross while they're running and you're walking to work eating a pastry (giving you that little guilt rush) are not a different species from you. They're probably enjoying their run as much as you're enjoying your snack. And for the same reason: an endorphin rush.

Endorphins are hormones our bodies release during pleasurable activities, including a tasty meal, sex, exercise, a massage and even shopping. They work wonders in reducing stress, and pain, giving us an overall sense of wellbeing. If you can shift your pleasure from sugar to a nice run, or even a brisk walk, you immediately switch off the come-down of the carbohydrate rush and keep the endorphin buzz, which can last hours, setting you off on a much better start or continuation of your day.

You can then keep those endorphins going throughout the day with sex (masturbation, if it's easier for you), listening to music or any non-dietary entertainment, gradually disassociating the feel-good feeling from snacking.

MOVE BEYOND DEDICATED EXERCISE

We promised we would help you move in more ways than sending you to the gym or running. The first one is switching a few habits in your day:

- **Walk or cycle to work:** sitting (public transportation or your car) burns an average of 80 calories per hour. Walking to work will burn 210 calories. Cycling takes between 300 and 600 calories, depending on effort and speed.

- **NEAT**, which stands for non-exercise activity thermogenesis, refers to every calorie burnt in simply getting on with your life. You can easily switch this one up by taking the stairs instead of the lift, getting away from your desk to make tea, picking up your lunch from the deli nearby, playing with your children for an extra 10 minutes, volunteering to take out the rubbish, and so on. While these changes won't individually mean much, being aware will make you more prone to act. Once they add up at the end of the day, you'll notice the difference.

BUILD YOUR MUSCLES

Cardiovascular exercise is associated with immediate calorie burn. When you run, cycle, dance or walk, your muscles are working – and consuming the calories. The higher the muscle mass, the higher the calorie expenditure to make them move. Dedicating time to increasing your muscle mass will make your movement more efficient. In addition to decreasing your body fat, an increased muscle mass will strengthen your immune system and energy levels and promote stress, anxiety and depression reduction.

MIND THE SPINE

Movement isn't only about calories and maintaining a healthy weight. It's a crucial aspect in supporting your spine, the connector of the central nervous system, the connecting hub of all bodily functions: mechanical, chemical and emotional.

The spine is a complex structure of bones, muscles and ligaments that shields the central nervous system, while allowing for movement and making us stand on our feet.

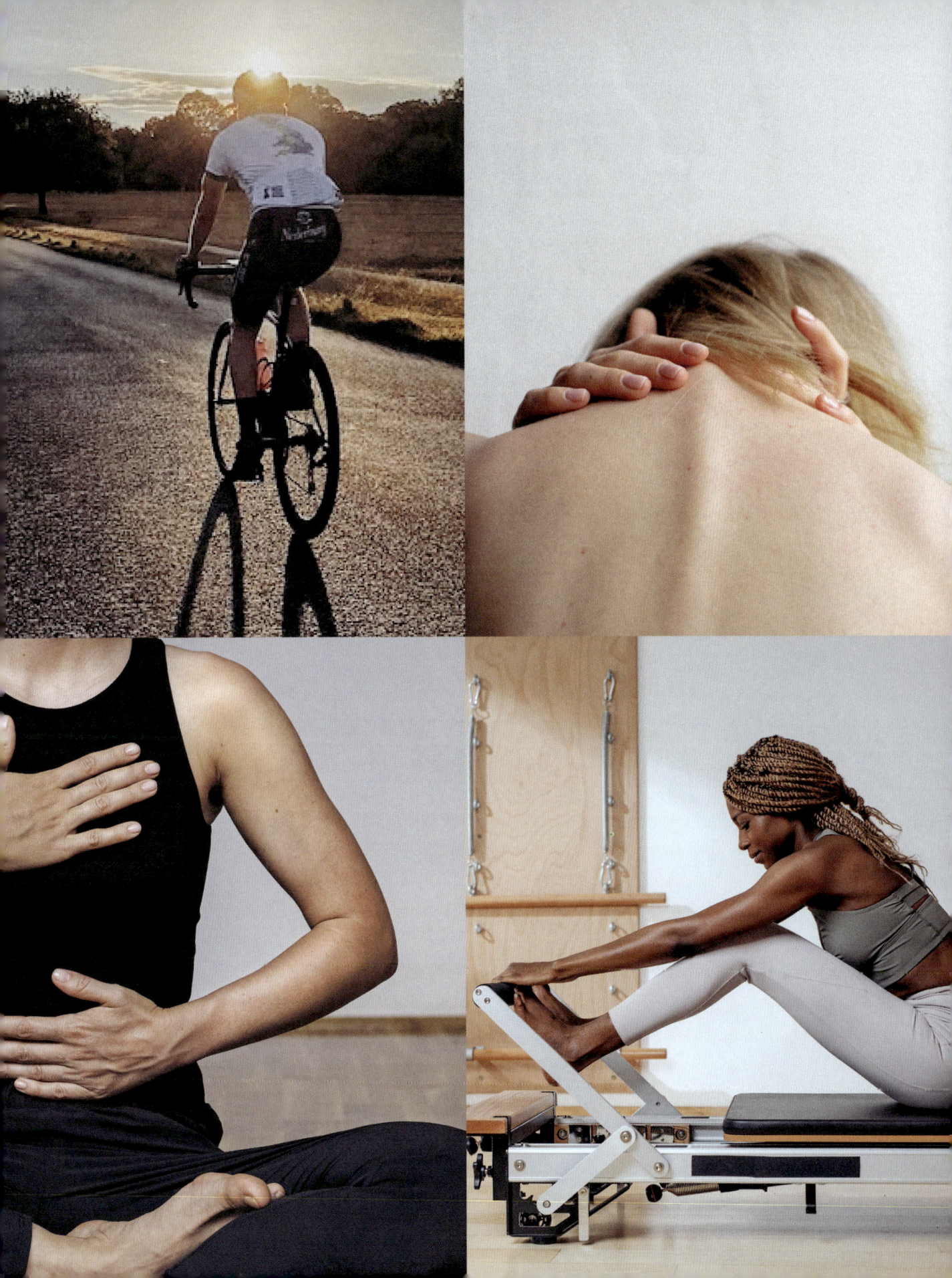

The spine consists of 33 bones stacked, protected and cushioned by the facet joints, which also promote spine movement. This impressive structure is, unsurprisingly, fragile. It's estimated that 80 per cent of people will experience back pain at some point in their lives, a number we should take seriously.

Good spine maintenance is about posture, which keeps our vertebrae aligned, and movement, which keeps the muscles and joints protecting the spine healthy and active.

anatomē's
STEPS FOR A HEALTHIER SPINE

Mind your posture
You can reduce everyday impact on your spine by teaching yourself better posture. Assess your desk for ergonomy – you want to have your feet on the ground and sit up straight.

Stretch
Sitting down – often in the wrong positions and for extended periods – will cause stiffness and miseducate your spine. Remember to stretch after sitting down for more than an hour, releasing the tension in the muscles and joints.

Keep moving
The spine produces four main types of movement: flexion, extension, rotation and lateral flexion. Keeping your spine in motion with exercise and an active daily life, minding the range of your movement, is fundamental to keeping your spine healthy and pain free.

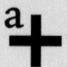

RECOVERY TIME

While we told you to keep moving to be healthier, recovery is necessary to give you control of the effects of good movement without overloading your body. After a high-intensity workout, the muscles will likely be inflamed and sore, with small tears due to the strain you've put them through. Your workout recovery will vary in length, depending on your fitness level, objectives, age and exercise intensity. Allowing 24–72 hours for your body to feel ready for another long session will help you build muscle, extend your movement range and avoid the long-term consequences of excess strain. Here are a few ways to help your muscles recover after a movement session:

HYDRATE

Restore your water and minerals after a workout with fresh water. It will help you cool down immediately after the session. In the following hours, the salts and the water will improve the recovery function, getting your muscles ready for the next workout quicker.

USE HEAT

Heat therapy is an efficient way of helping your body recover after an intense workout session (according to research, up to 47 per cent if done 24 hours post-exercise). A warm (not too hot) bath or shower enriched with bath salts will dilate your blood vessels, increasing the blood flow to the muscles and relaxing them. The improved circulation will help oxygen reach the muscles, along with the nutrients needing replenishment. A warm session will also help you get rid of accumulated lactic acid. Lactic acid, produced during intense exercise, causes muscle fatigue and soreness. While lactic acid can improve endurance, it must be eliminated to avoid lactic acidosis, which builds up in the muscles and bloodstream, leading to symptoms such as nausea and vomiting.

USE ICE (IF YOU NEED TO)

Cold therapy, also known as cryotherapy, is needed in case of an injury – even if a minor one. It works by reducing the blood flow to the injured muscle or joint, reducing bruising and pain. Apply cold water or ice to an injured region immediately after the event to reduce soreness and slow down any inflammation.

anatomē's
GUIDE TO CREATING THE PERFECT BATH

Baths are the most intimate moment we can spend with ourselves. Extending them and creating habits to enhance this time can make them one of the most potent antidotes to the stress of the outside world.

Here's how to do it:

Create a mood. Light a candle to fill your bathroom with your favourite scents, dim or adjust the lighting, remove any screens from sight and keep your skin and haircare on hand. Remember to leave your towel and bathrobe ready for when you finish your practice. This may seem like a list of chores, but they'll become second nature once you discover the pleasures of a good bath. Add gentle music to help set the mood and keep external noise away.

Mind the temperature. While the temperature of your bath is a personal choice, staying close to 40°C (104°F) is recommended to avoid damaging your skin with heat. Starting at a slightly higher temperature and letting it cool to the ideal level is fine.

Add salts. Adding salts to your bath can reduce internal swelling, moisturize the skin, detoxify the body and relax the muscles thanks to the minerals in them, which are absorbed by the skin from the hot water and get into the bloodstream.

Apply an essential oil. The steam is a natural expectorant, helping to open your airways and allowing your body receive the scent – making more of each drop you use.

Relax. Take the time to breathe, practise mindfulness and focus on your self-care.

Leave the bath gently. Allow for post-bath time, avoiding rushing through drying, rinsing and getting ready. The last thing you need is to undo the good work of bathing mindfully by getting back into stress mode.

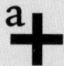

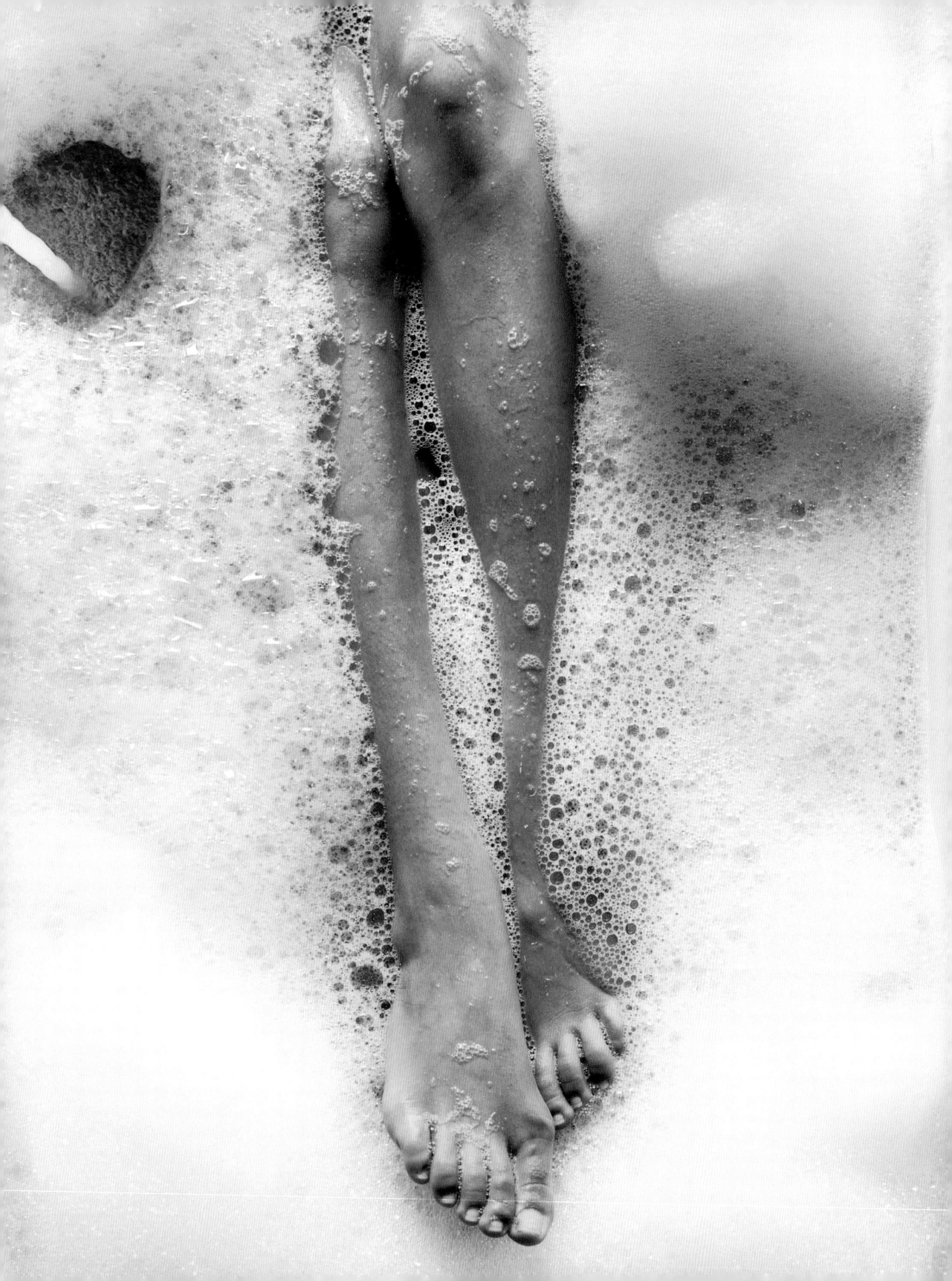

EXERCISE THROUGH THE AGES

Exercise has always been a key tenet of good health and wellbeing. From the ancient Greeks to the Victorians, good physical fitness was considered the mark of an upstanding citizen and, collectively, of a strong society.

Ancient Greece

For the young men of ancient Greece, the gymnasium was a part of their education. Anacharsis, a Scythian philosopher from the Black Sea area and traveller who visited Greece, famously said: 'In every Greek city, there is one place they go mad daily, which I mean to be the gymnasium.' This activity may have seemed strange to both ancient and modern observers, however, for the Greeks, exercise was an essential aspect of what we now refer to as wellbeing. The ancient Greek historian Diodorus even claimed that gymnasia and temples promoted happiness.

The ancient Greeks understood that to achieve and maintain wellness, diet alone wouldn't cut it: they needed to exercise. Hippocrates, the Greek father of medicine, insisted that good eating alone could not keep a person well. Fitness and health were also esteemed, visible characteristics in Grecian culture; athletes were often depicted unclothed in artwork as exemplifying moral worth. The term 'gymnasium' originates from *gymnos*, Greek for 'naked', recognizing nudity as a representation of heroic virtue.

Ancient Rome

Hippocrates may have laid the groundwork for Greek medicine, but it was the Roman Galen who made significant strides in the field. As a physician, writer and philosopher, he took what Hippocrates had established and built a more comprehensive understanding of the human body, particularly during physical exertion.

He observed: 'In my view, movement alone isn't necessarily deemed exercise; rather it must be vigorous to be considered as such. It should be noted that what is vigorous for one person may not be as intense for another.' He even went on to observe that, although it's impossible to prevent ageing altogether, regular exercise can certainly slow down its onset.

The Renaissance

The Renaissance was a period of not only intellectual revival but physical too. Vittorino da Feltre, an Italian humanist, initiated the trend in 1420 by setting up an institution with a focus on physical education. Mercuriale's *De Arte Gymnastica*, released in 1569, was one of the initial works to examine the therapeutic aspects of exercise and recreational activities.

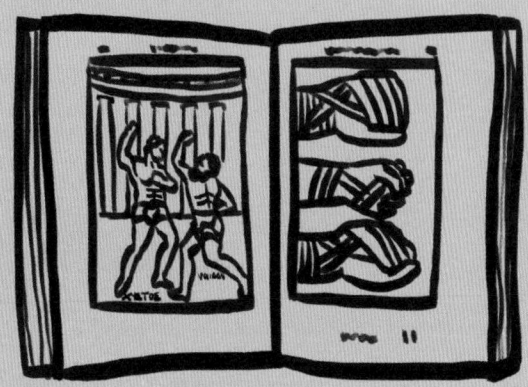

1800s

From the early nineteenth century, there was a desire to promote physical exercise to balance out factory life. That led to the invention of machines that could facilitate activity – and one of the most well-known inventions was the bicycle, created by German civil servant Baron Karl von Drais in 1817. However, it wasn't until the development of the so-called 'safety bicycle' in the 1880s and 1890s that bicycles became accessible to all genders, ages and economic backgrounds. Where usage had previously been limited to wealthy, leisurely individuals, these developments allowed cycling to become a widespread means of transportation.

The birth of nineteenth-century ideas of nationalism led to the idea of physical fitness as embodying not just personal health but that of the nation – influenced too by Darwin's 'survival of the fittest'. To be fit and healthy was, once again, in an echo of ancient Greece, to be an upstanding citizen. And for the first time, women became part of this movement, representing their countries at the Olympic Games alongside men – although in smaller numbers.

1900s

As the twentieth century progressed, physical education for children grew in importance, especially in Germany, where Prussia had implemented a gymnastics curriculum in 1862. The concept of 'fitness' took a turn with the Nazi vision. In 1937, 'gym' classes for boys were introduced in state schools. But, rather than health reasons, it was part of the build-up of dark times: it was about moulding strong Aryan bodies for the imminent war.

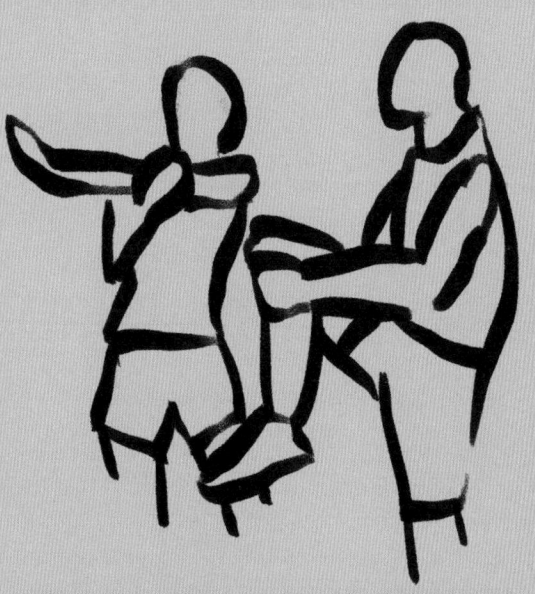

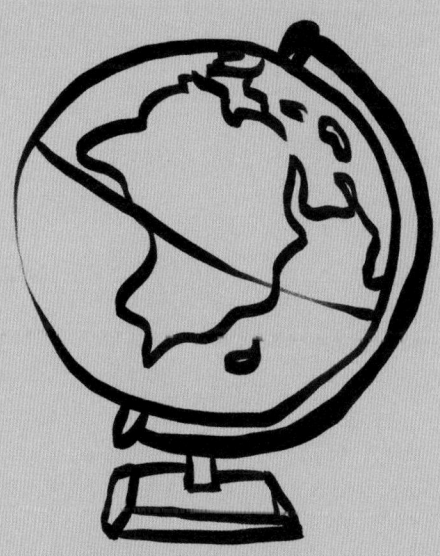

Today

Physical activity is a normal part of life for many around the world, from school PE classes to global sporting events. The evidence for its many benefits accumulates, improving our physical and mental wellbeing.

anatomē believes in the power of physical activity to improve our emotions, relax muscles and quieten anxious minds. Recent research has identified how it stimulates changes in the brain – confirming the idea of the 'runner's high'.

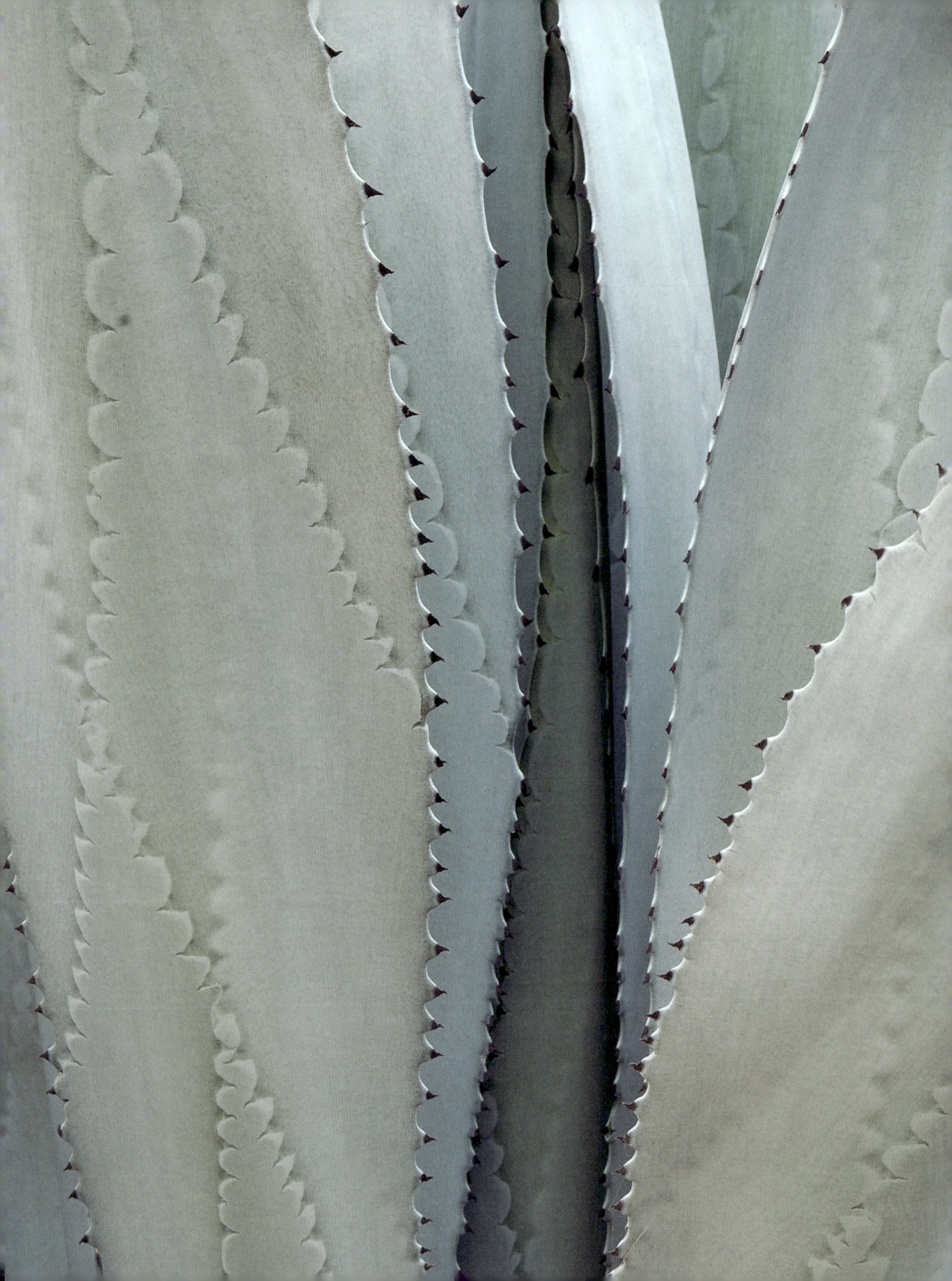

4
FOCUS

What it is and how it works

Focusing refers to the ability to concentrate on mental or physical activity. It's relative, depending on the type of activity, expectations and expected outcome, which makes it challenging to assess collectively. At anatomē, we discuss focus individually, listening to our community members' challenges and expectations.

Most of us, at some level, face challenges with focusing. Whether it's getting through a work task, preparing for an interview or even getting our lives organized, distraction or detachment from an activity is natural and an increasing situation in modern living.

Focus deficit has different causes. If you struggle with it, the first step you need to take to tackle it is to identify your type of focus deficit. One of them is your attention span, which is the length of time you can concentrate on an activity or subject. The other is concentration, which refers to the mental effort level you dedicate to something – regardless of how long for.

FACTORS THAT AFFECT CONCENTRATION

Whether your challenge is concentration or attention span, the good news is that focus deficit is highly influenced by external and internal factors that you can control. anatomē believes in identifying them and their causes and then training your mind to refocus.

In this assessment, we will aim to identify the root of your focus challenge, not the distractions or excuses. Our goal is to improve your ability to focus, not blame yourself for losing it in the first place. For instance, it's easy to blame social media or your phone for your struggle to finish a work presentation. What about determining why you're reaching for it instead of keeping your mind on the job?

INCORRECT DIET AND NUTRITION

Bingeing on sugary treats or going on a 'miracle' weight-loss diet without seeking specialist advice can affect your concentration. Low-fat diets, for instance, may deprive your brain of essential fatty acids. Protein is also essential as a source of the amino acids that create the chemicals your brain uses to focus.

Then let's not forget the vitamins B and D and minerals such as iron: all of which will determine how well your brain will work – directly affecting your focus.

Whether due to dieting or skipping meals for a time, hunger is another terrible distraction for the brain. The loss of energy from low blood sugar is one of the brain's worst enemies, immediately affecting your ability to pay attention.

DEHYDRATION

Studies have proven that a dehydrated body has a lower ability to focus. Hangovers are a clear example. After a big night out involving alcohol, we tend to have a write-off day for mental and physical productivity. Some call that a hangover, but the root of the problem is sheer dehydration. Our brains are so sensitive to lack of water, even a 1 per cent below recommended hydration level can affect our focus.

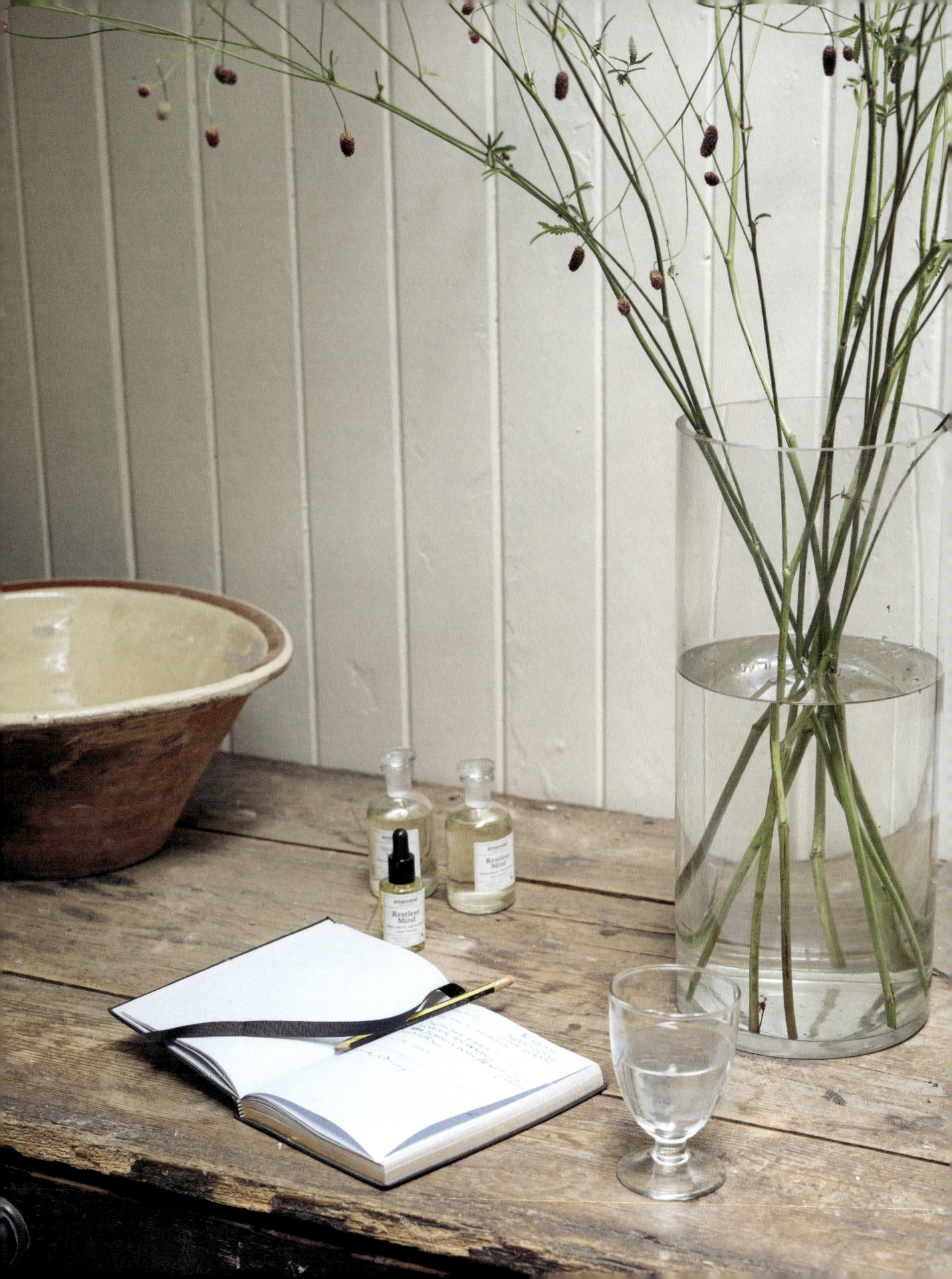

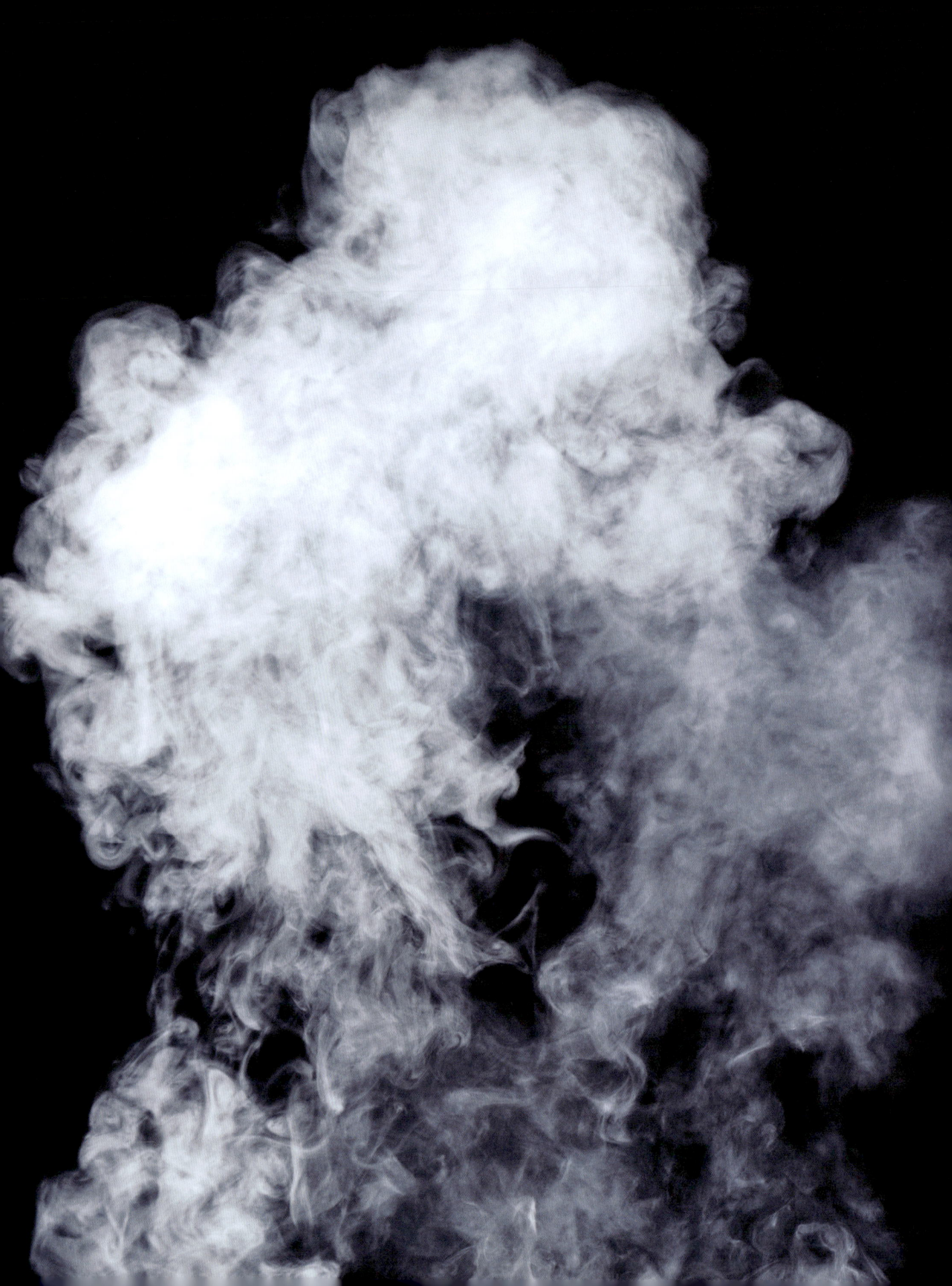

HORMONAL CHANGES

Hormonal fluctuation – particularly in women – is another focus killer. It's not unusual for women to mention feeling a little airheaded during pregnancy – a frequent symptom known commonly as 'baby brain', with various manifestations including forgetfulness, difficulties in keeping up with work tasks and brain fog.

Meanwhile, loss of concentration is one of the many symptoms of menopause, acknowledged by physicians and experienced by many women going through this life change.

LACK OF SLEEP

Not getting enough sleep, or not sleeping restfully enough, will make you less alert and drastically affect your focus. In severe cases, more than two nights of insufficient sleep can send someone on a worrying journey of lack of focus, negativity and stress.

Over time, while the body may get somewhat accustomed to sleeping less, the brain will work under a chronic concentration deficit, making someone consistently unfocused. If you label yourself 'flaky', 'distracted' or 'unfocused', the sleep chapter of this book may reveal you're simply not sleeping well enough.

STRESS

The feeling of freezing under stress is not unusual. The longer your to-do list, the more difficult it seems to tackle. You may even reach out to your phone and completely switch off, mindlessly watching reels until an internal alarm tells you it's time to get back to work. You get back to work but forget what was on the list, the priorities and not knowing where to begin. Add that to mindless reading – the kind that has you re-reading the same page because you haven't retained what you just read.

That is because continuous stress – emotional, professional or health-related – triggers short circuits in our cognitive functions.

MEDICAL AND PSYCHOLOGICAL PROBLEMS

Focus deficit may also be a symptom of a health condition, manifesting in patients with ongoing conditions such as sleep apnoea, visual issues, early-onset dementia, brain injury, depression, anxiety and traumas alike. If you worry about this being your case, it's imperative to seek a medical assessment and treat the medical condition before anything else.

SEDENTARISM

Studies have shown that, after 3 months of aerobic exercise, individuals have shown improvements in neuroplasticity – the brain's ability to form and reorganize synaptic connections and create new neurons. On the other hand, not moving enough may deprive your brain of the chance of growing, developing and keeping in shape.

YOUR ENVIRONMENT

This is the first one we blame. Too noisy, too dark, too hot and so on are the most blamed factors for lack of concentration. And we're right to do so. If your workspace isn't correctly set up to promote focus, it can impact your performance. If you work at a desk, ergonomic factors should also be assessed (lighting, chair, desk height, computer placement and so on). If you are constantly interrupted by colleagues, family or anyone around you, consider that an environmental factor, too.

QUALITY OF INFORMATION

Incorrect information, vague emails, passive-aggressive messages, excess images and bad work culture result in low-quality material to work with. As such, our brains tend to reject the content we're assessing, switching off and making us lose our focus. If you roll your eyes at one in every three emails you receive and start online shopping while pretending to be attending a call, it may be because you're surrounded by people who work at a lower level than you expect. (Did you finish the last sentence in your head with a term for them? We did, too, at first.)

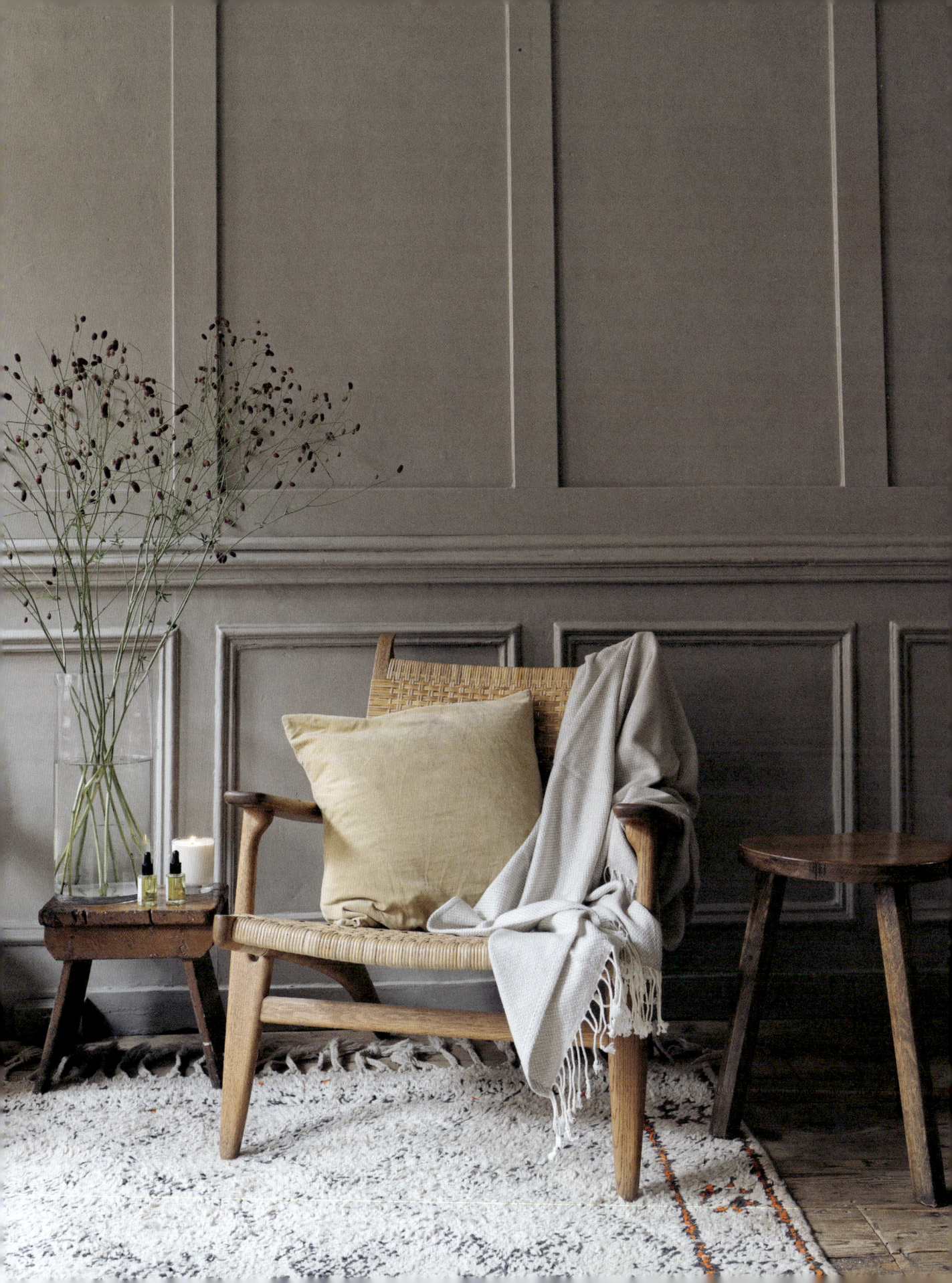

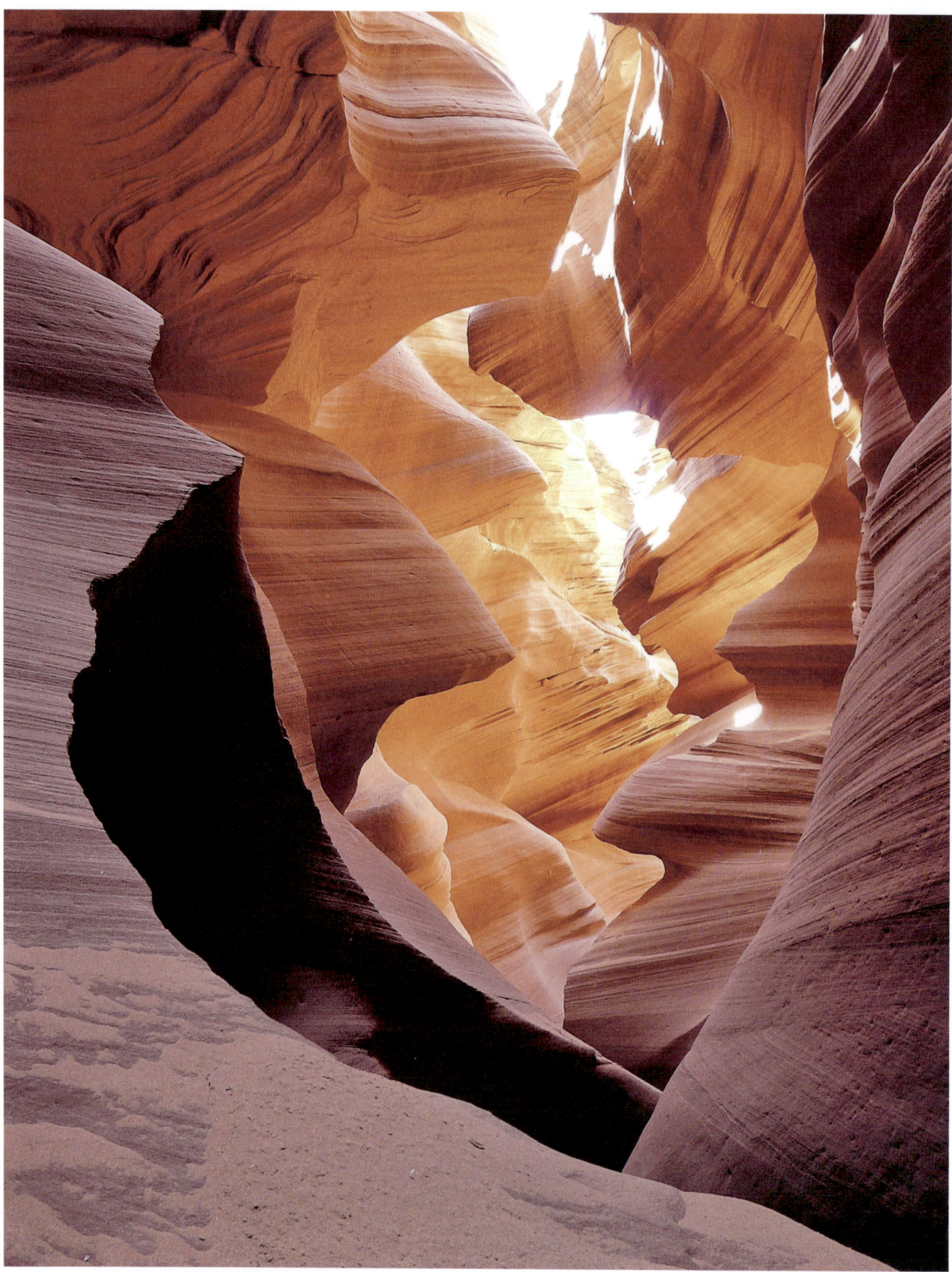

HOW TO IMPROVE YOUR FOCUS

After you've identified the cause – or causes – of your focus deficit, it's time to consider what steps you can take to regain your focus. It's important to know that wellbeing pillars work combined. As such, you'll likely touch other aspects of your lifestyle make-up to switch up your concentration.

MINDFULNESS

According to neuropsychologist Kim Willment, 'Mindfulness is about focusing attention on the present moment, and practising mindfulness has been shown to rewire the brain so that attention is stronger in everyday life.' A few daily minutes, preferably with your eyes closed and focus directed to your breathing and bodily sensations, will make a good start. Later in this book, we will discuss the details of mindfulness and how you can train your brain to be more mindful.

COGNITIVE TRAINING

Cognitive training exercises often involve pattern detection, memorizing lists and absorbing new information.

There are simple and easy-to-get-into ways of training your brain's cognitive function. Some of them, such as baking, learning a new language or taking drawing lessons, may take too much effort and time (although a new hobby can be game-changing in supporting your wellbeing, see page 67).

You can find easy solutions online or via apps. They include memory games, word scrabble, Tetris and other concentration games that can easily take up some of your mindless social-media-scrolling time, converting it into brain-training minutes and improving your focus. If you want to train your mind while avoiding screens, a good solution is puzzles, crosswords and sudoku in print versions – an excellent way to unwind away from blue lights from electronic devices. Blue light from electronic devices can suppress the production of melatonin, a hormone that regulates sleep-wake cycles. Exposure to blue light in the evening or at night can disrupt circadian rhythms, making it harder to fall asleep and reducing sleep quality.

EMBRACE FOCUS-SUPPORTING INGREDIENTS

You can power your focus practices with a dose of ingredients selected for their proven benefits to the brain. For instance, lion's mane and cordyceps – which are types of fungi – are examples of powerful ingredients often used in supplements. These mushrooms support the generation of ATP, the energy molecule, optimizing brain cell metabolism and protection from short- and long-term cell ageing. They stimulate brain activity, generate energy for the body and brain and maintain brain cell signalling and impulse transmission – resulting in better memory performance and concentration.

Embrace the power of scent and switch your brain on with essential oil formulations made up of invigorating ingredients that support clarity of thought and cognitive performance, as well as relieving mental fatigue, such as Indian ginger root, cinnamon and frankincense. Look for versions rich in terpene oils for the ultimate awakening blend to alleviate stress and support clear thought processes, creativity and focus. For more on terpenes, see page 170.

MAKE CHANGES TO YOUR WORK ENVIRONMENT

Invest in new lighting, an appropriate chair and desk, laptop-supporting equipment and any other elements necessary to make your work environment more comfortable. You may want to assess the noise levels and the distractions you currently face while working – if you can – and make sure you're properly geared and accommodated to perform.

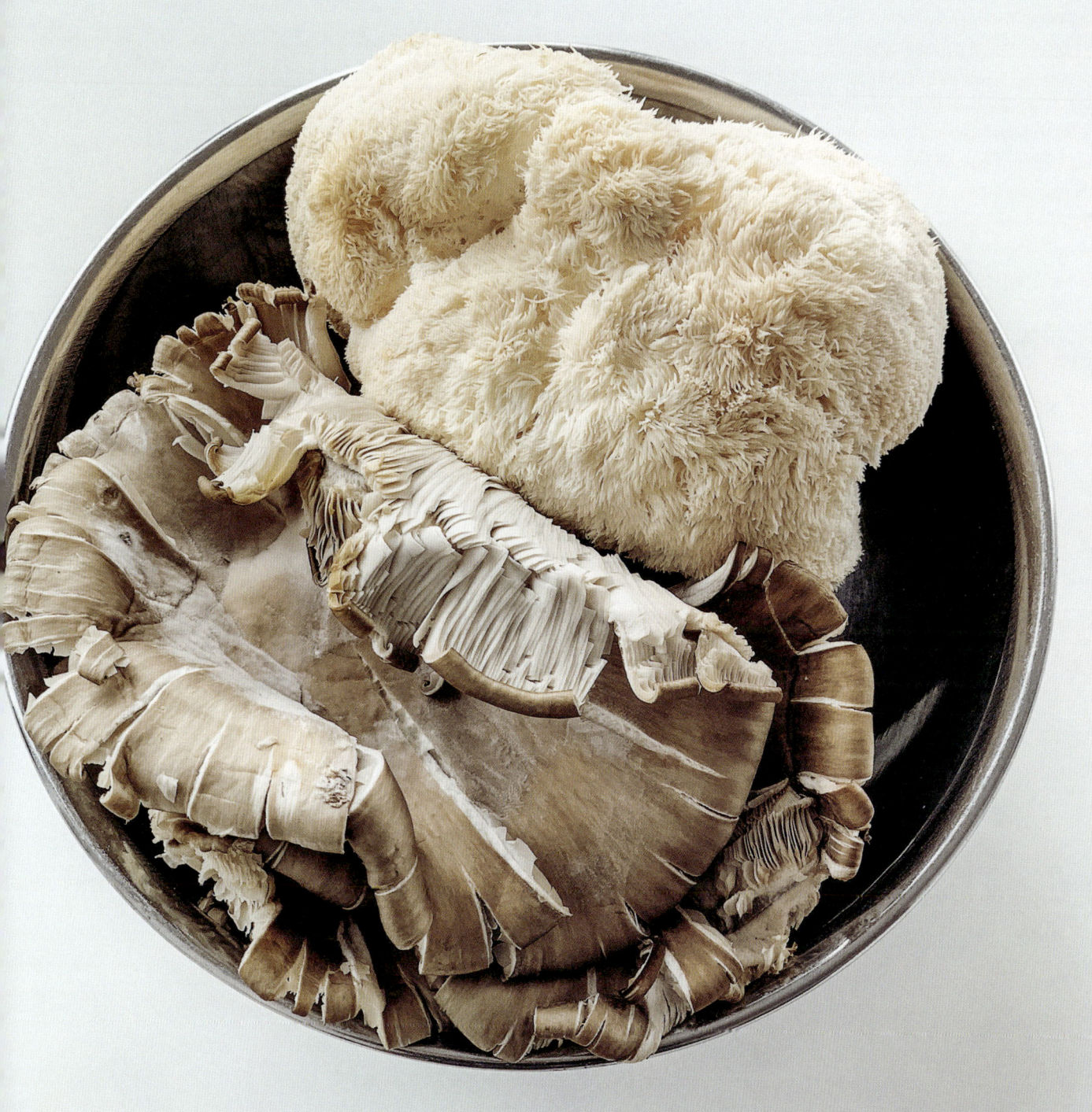

5
DIET

Eat well to live well is an old saying. We know about the benefits of a healthy diet to our physical health. We grow up learning the basics of a good diet, the nutritional importance of some foods, what to avoid to prevent disease, and even how to keep our weight in check.

Then come the diet trends and fads we tap into when we feel like getting into shape or shedding a few pounds. In between diets, we indulge in food and drink, succumb to the pleasures of fat, sugar, alcohol and carbohydrates, throwing food balance out the window. And then we regret our behaviour.

But the importance of a good, balanced diet goes beyond simply maintaining a healthy weight. Recent studies have shown that upholding good gut health influences wellbeing much more directly than we imagined.

Let's support this conversation with facts. Our digestive system does far more than process the food and drink we consume, converting it into energy and producing waste. We have an entire nervous system within our digestive tract. Scientists call it the enteric nervous system (ENS).

The ENS consists of 100 million nerve cells. They're lining our entire gastrointestinal tract – from the oesophagus to the rectum. And they communicate directly with our brains.

Brain-to-gut communications aren't emotional or rational but functional and involuntary. It's a control system of numerous operations that regulates the intake, conversion and utilization of the fuel we feed our bodies into the energy we use to keep those bodies alive. And then informs how and when to discard the waste of this operation.

For years, we believed gut problems such as irritable bowel syndrome (IBS), constipation, diarrhoea, bloating and pain could be bodily reactions to mental health issues such as depression and anxiety. Recent studies have shown that, in many cases, it all starts in the gut: researchers found that gastrointestinal conditions trigger messages to the central nervous system, which in turn affects our mood.

While these studies are under development, these findings add a compelling new reason to maintain a good diet and prioritize gut health when looking after our wellbeing.

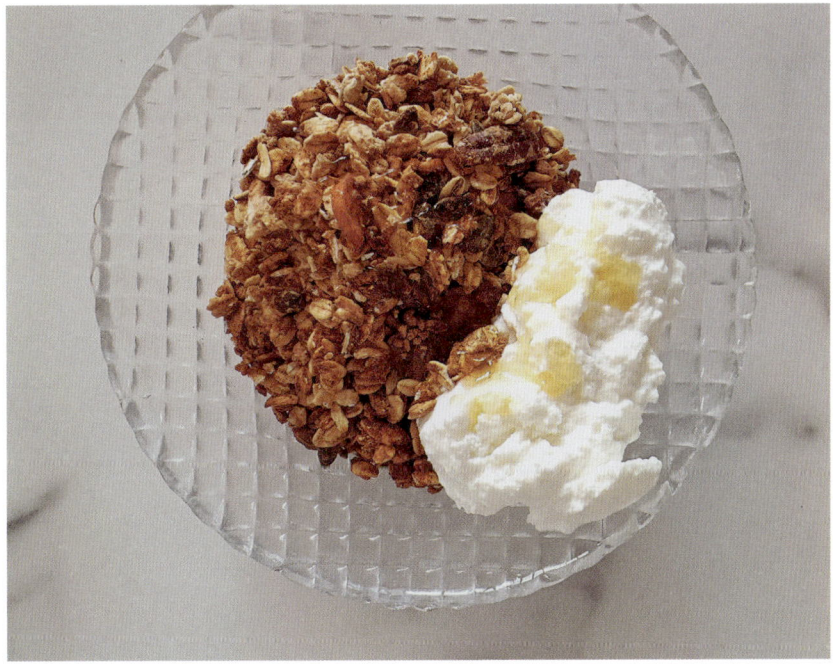

DIETS THROUGH THE AGES

The term 'diet' has evolved over time. Originally meaning the total consumed amount of food and drink, it now often refers to restricting food intake to lose weight or change physical appearance. This shift has been brought about by modern food preservation and transportation, enabling people to consume more options than just what they could find or hunt from the land.

700–480 BC

Ancient Greece was the first civilization to popularize ideas of fitness and healthy eating, although their definition of an 'ideal' body was not focused on looks, but on physical, athletic abilities.

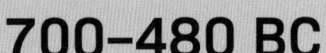

1500s

Since 1558, the notion of 'ideal body types' has been around, with Luigi Cornaro's *The Art of Living Long* being the first diet book still in print today. It urges readers to limit food intake and consume wine. This prompted *The Fruits, Herbs and Vegetables of Italy* by Giacomo Castelvetro, which became the basis for today's celebrated Mediterranean Diet. A century later, Dr George Cheyne wrote *The Natural Method of Curing the Diseases of the Body, and Diseases of the Mind, Depending on the Body*, detailing his exclusively vegetable and dairy diet.

500–1000 AD

In medieval Europe, the idea of a balanced diet, known as *regimen sanitatis*, gained prominence, focusing on moderation, variety and seasonal eating. One landmark in the history of diets was the influential work of Galen, a Roman physician whose writings on food and diet greatly influenced medical and dietary practices throughout the medieval period.

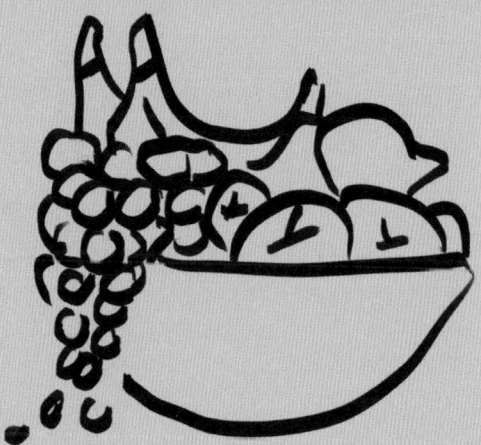

1800s

In the mid-1800s, Lord Byron gained renown as a 'diet influencer' due to his attractive appearance and famous vinegar diet – where he drank vinegar with water and ate potatoes soaked in it. People began to follow his lead, but to their peril; there are records of individuals dying from ingesting too much vinegar.

The thin, frail figure of the Victorian era was made iconic by Empress Elisabeth Amalie Wittelsbach, also known as Sisi. To stay slender, she went on long walks, rode horses, did gymnastics and abstained from eating much.

The first low-carb diet was introduced in *The Physiology of Taste or Meditations on Transcendental Gastronomy* by Jean Anthelme Brillat-Savarin in 1825. This work set a precedent against perceiving obesity as an illness, but, instead, as a result of one's lifestyle. It suggested avoiding carbohydrate-rich food such as bread and potatoes.

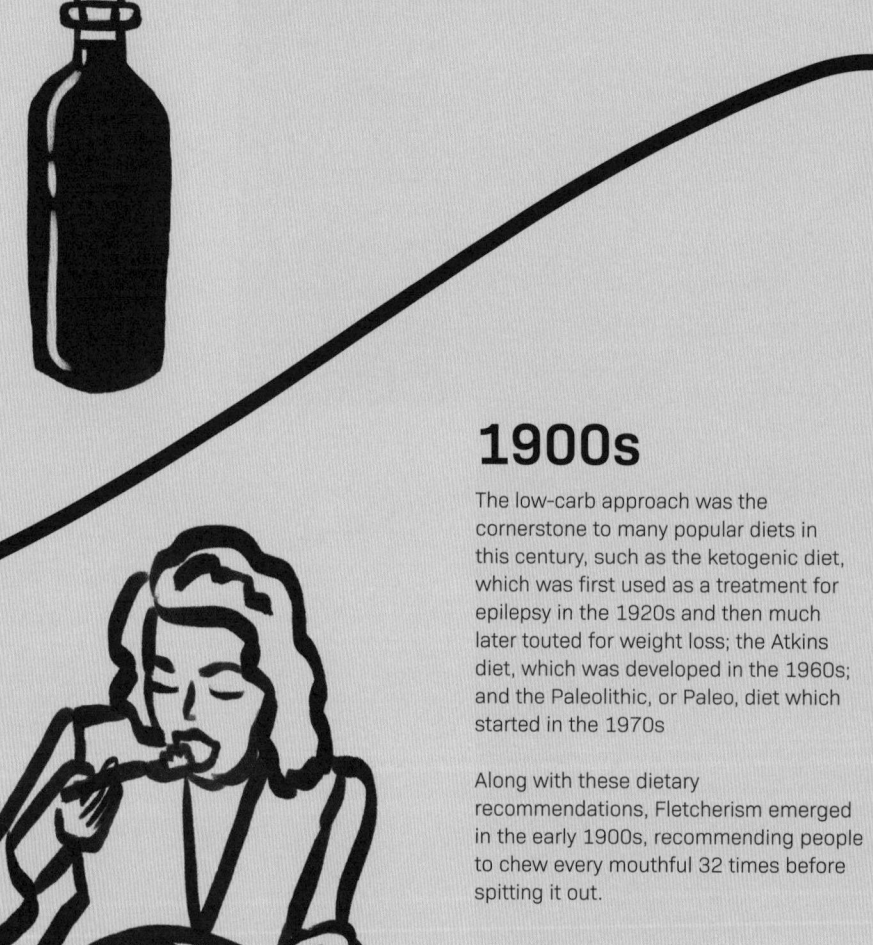

1900s

The low-carb approach was the cornerstone to many popular diets in this century, such as the ketogenic diet, which was first used as a treatment for epilepsy in the 1920s and then much later touted for weight loss; the Atkins diet, which was developed in the 1960s; and the Paleolithic, or Paleo, diet which started in the 1970s

Along with these dietary recommendations, Fletcherism emerged in the early 1900s, recommending people to chew every mouthful 32 times before spitting it out.

2000s

In the first decade of the twenty-first century, dietary trends evolved rapidly, with a celebrity-driven influence. Concepts of diet expanded to include sustainability, ethics and personalization. Plant-based diets fuelled by celebrity endorsements gained mainstream popularity, while organic and local foods gained traction. Online platforms and social media amplified dietary information, shaping wellness practices.

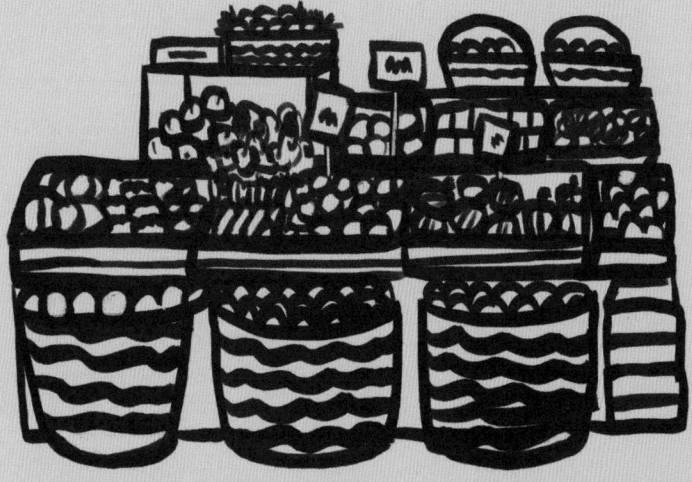

2010s

The concept of dieting has changed within popular culture. Rather than its original definition, it now often refers to ways in which people restrict the amount of food they consume. Social media and pop culture have only heightened the presence of diet fads – juice cleanses and liquid diets, for example. If you want to manage your weight, patience and dietary education are the only safe way. It's still more efficient to rely on a healthy, varied diet combined with regular exercise as a path to health and wellbeing.

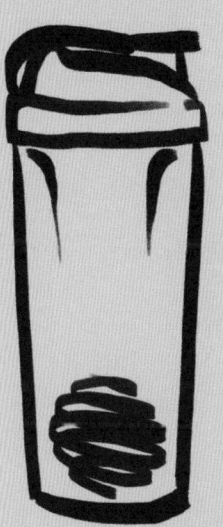

THE BENEFITS OF A HEALTHY GUT

Let's begin by clarifying what we mean by 'healthy gut', removing any disambiguation and focusing our plan to get yours on track if needed. Our gut, or gastrointestinal tract, is filled with bacteria – good and bad. We call this colony the gut microbiome. The 'good' bacteria help control harmful bacteria by multiplying vigorously and often, stunting the growth of the unhealthy kind. This delicate balance within the gut is called equilibrium.

Without equilibrium, the body is in danger. Studies have found that excess harmful bacteria in the gut can cause day-to-day discomfort and make us prone to developing Crohn's disease, ulcerative colitis and irritable bowel syndrome (IBS), along with other conditions. A healthy gut has higher levels of good bacteria in the microbiome, functioning harmoniously to regulate any effect of harmful organisms. By 'harmoniously', we mean reduced inflammatory elements that lead to coronary disease, cancer and autoimmune diseases.

But the benefits of a healthy gut don't stop there. A healthy gut will:

- Strengthen your immune system.
- Improve brain health.
- Lift your mood and help keep depression and anxiety at bay.
- Support healthy sleep.

Our entire bodies receive signals from the brain. And the gut might rebel at times. According to studies, the balance of bacteria in our gut microbiome may influence our emotions and how our brain interprets information from the senses, such as sights, sounds, flavours or sensations. Changes in that equilibrium may contribute to disorders like anxiety and depression, as well as chronic pain.

Bacteria also affect our ability to maintain a healthy diet. Incorrect messages from our brains about feeling hungry or full may result from an unbalanced gut microbiota. The pituitary gland, which produces hormones that help regulate appetite, is thought by researchers to be connected to the condition.

The gut microbes also influence the skin. Substance P is a neuropeptide produced in the gut, brain and skin, which plays a major role in skin conditions. An imbalanced gut microbiome promotes the release of substance P in both the gut and the skin.

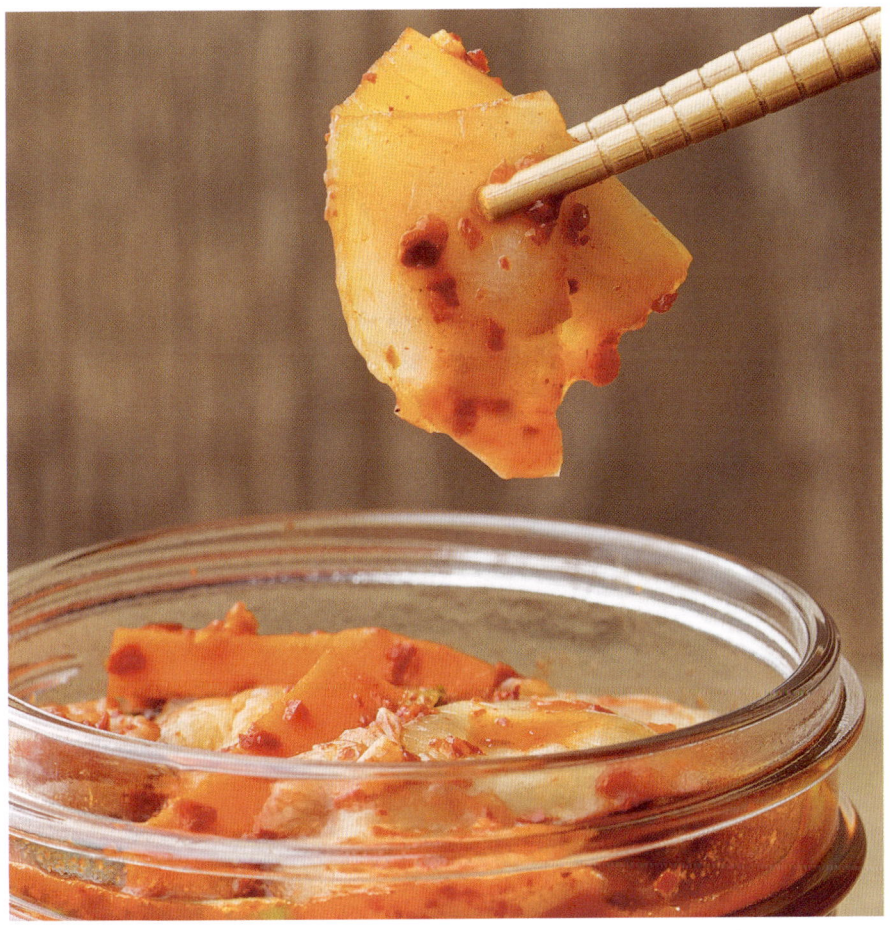

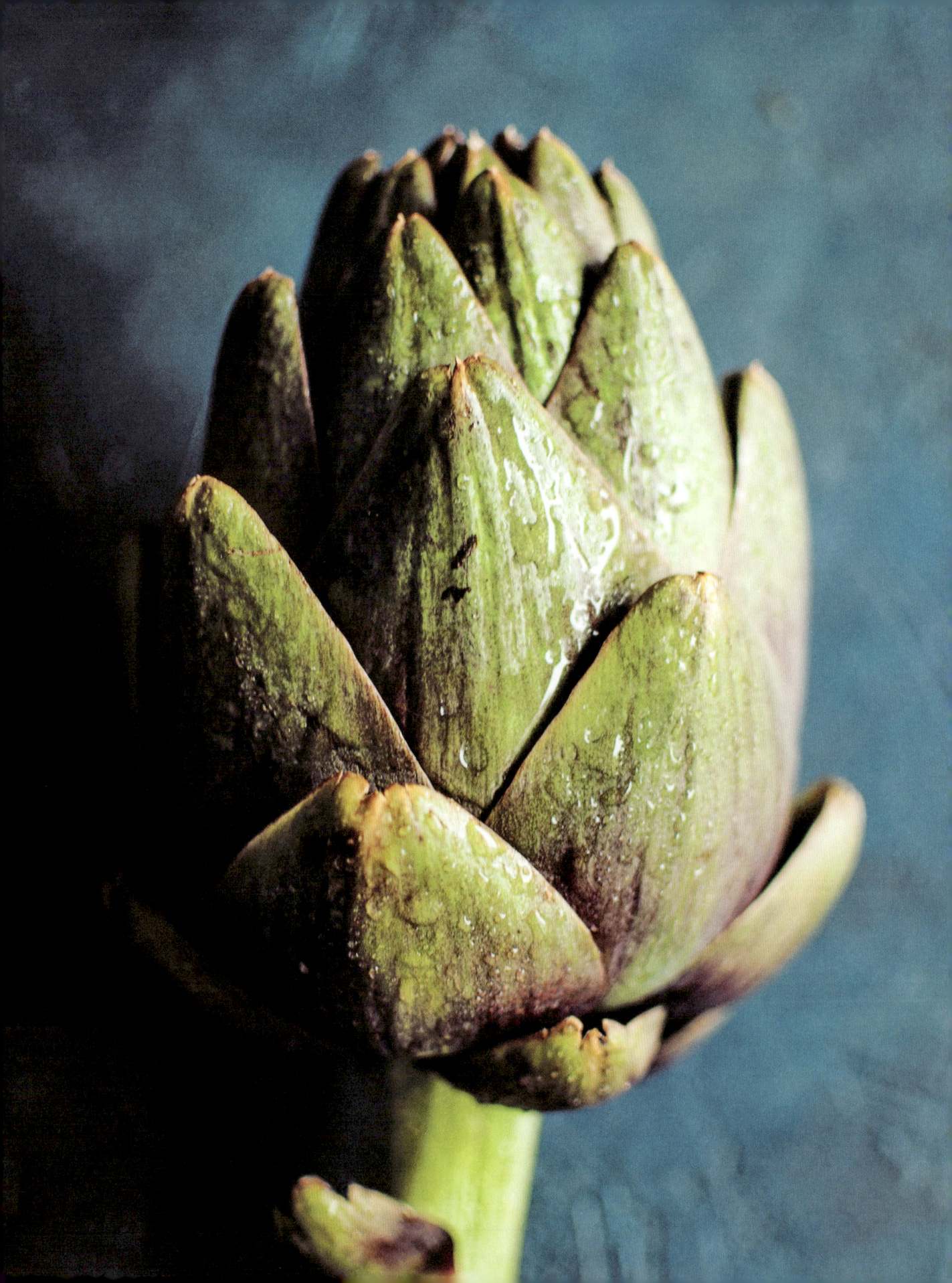

PROBIOTICS

Live bacteria, also known as probiotics or 'good' bacteria, may boost the intestinal tract's bacterial population and support the maintenance of proper gut balance. But they aren't all the same. Each kind functions uniquely and can have a variety of physiological impacts.

Probiotics can also make your gut stronger. They might improve digestive health, particularly if you suffer from irritable bowel syndrome. Certain probiotics may also assist with lactose intolerance and allergy problems. But because everyone's gut flora differs, it can vary whether and how they function. Further research on that front is under development.

Sources of probiotics

We can find probiotics in dairy products such as aged cheeses and yoghurt. When shopping, check for live cultures of bacteria like bifidobacteria and lactobacilli on the ingredients list. They're also present in pickled vegetables like onions and gherkins, and fermented vegetables like kimchi and sauerkraut.

Prebiotics are also a food source for probiotics. They help our bodies absorb calcium better and boost the growth of good bacteria. We can find them in fruits and vegetables such as bananas, onions, garlic, leeks, asparagus, artichokes, soya and any food produced with whole wheat.

The benefits of oral probiotics

These have been shown to decrease the gut permeability, improving the intestinal barrier function and reducing inflammation. They also decrease the production of pro-inflammatory cytokines within the skin, improving its condition.

Oral and topical probiotics reduce systemic markers of inflammation and oxidative stress, elevated locally in those with acne. Oxidative stress is the imbalance between producing reactive oxygen species (ROS) – molecules that can cause damage to cells, tissues and DNA – and the body's ability to detoxify or neutralize them with antioxidants. High quantities of operating ROS can cause damage to cellular membranes, proteins, and DNA, potentially contributing to the development of various diseases, including cancer, diabetes, cardiovascular disease and neurodegenerative disorders.

WELLBEING VILLAINS

So we have talked pillars, but before we revisit healing with wellbeing practices, let's talk – briefly, we promise – about some of our most dreaded villains: feelings, mindsets and symptoms that we must learn to fight to preserve our wellness.

Before you turn the page to find out what they are (you've already done that, haven't you?), you should know you're likely to be suffering with some – if not all of them – daily.

You're not alone. Read through each feeling carefully, identify your causes, and practice awareness to help you manage them, or at least be aware if they come to haunt you.

These aren't the only ones, but they are the most widely identifiable causes of stress, undoing the good work we do on building our wellbeing and happiness. Knowing them is the first step to overcoming them.

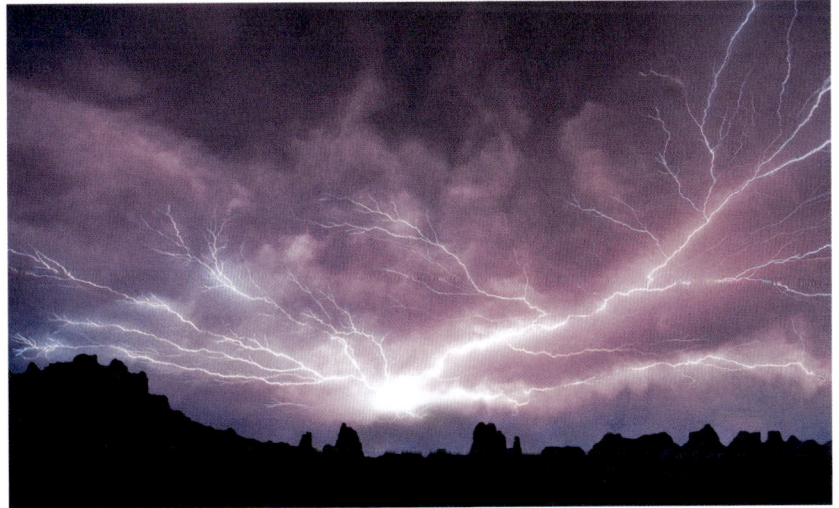

1 FOMO – FEAR OF MISSING OUT

We first heard of FoMO in 2004. It came from a marketing technique to drive urgency in people, pushing them to shop by triggering an anxious, often irrational urgency feeling in their brains.

Then, with the advent of social networking, in 2010, we began to apply this expression to a new, terrifying feeling that life is happening somewhere other than around us. And we aren't invited.

It describes what it says on the tin: 'Fear of Missing Out', and refers to the perception in itself and the compulsive behaviour to include ourselves, maintain relationships and make sure we're participating in everything presented to us.

Social media platforms, such as Instagram, provide us with a constant influx of information and images from the lives of others. While this can be entertaining and informative, it can also negatively affect our mental health as exposure to curated and retouched images of others' seemingly perfect lives can cause social media anxiety and lead to feelings of inadequacy.

This can be exacerbated by the rapid-fire scrolling and constant notifications, creating a sense of urgency and pressure to keep up. As a result, we may feel anxious, stressed or depressed, especially when comparing our lives to those we see online.

The exposure to multiple realities within fractions of a second subconsciously awakens negative life experiences, making us feel excluded and unworthy and harming our self-esteem.

anatomē's
STEPS FOR MANAGING FOMO

MAIN CAUSE: Excessive or problematic use of social media.

TREATMENT: We don't expect you to delete your social media, but there are some ways to make it less harmful.

1 Unfollow accounts, chat groups or any source of content that makes you feel anxious. If you can't unfollow an account for a specific reason (other than guilt, please), mute it.

2 Limit your social media and texting time, avoiding it in the first and last 2 hours of your day.

3 Create a gentle reminder for yourself of the parallel reality that social media is. Something funny and ironic that you can think about every time your FoMO flares up. You can even find content that unveils the truth behind social-media perfection, with bloopers and unretouched versions of images.

4 Establish a weekly social-media fasting time. It can be as short as 1 hour. Enjoy something physical or sensorial during this time. It can be a massage, a meal or exercise. Try to increase this weekly non-social media time, either in length or frequency.

5 Resist the urge to reply or react instantly to messages or social media posts. Whether something triggered anger, urgency or made you worry, you can – and should – take your time before you reply to refine the communication of your sentiment and train your body to accept challenges, while remaining serene.

2 WORKPLACE ANXIETY

Workplace anxiety is a reality. In a recent poll conducted by the American Psychological Association, nearly 40 per cent of Americans have reported feeling anxious at some point. In 2022, Beyoncé's single *Break My Soul*, in which the lyrics depict a typical case of workplace anxiety, resonated so well with her audience it reportedly motivated fans to quit their jobs.

We pay attention to such collective manifestations at anatomē, as they help us understand a global sentiment, inspiring our formulation process and new practices.

Often diagnosed as someone's 'normal' anxiety manifesting itself in the workplace, a specific type of anxiety related to any aspect of your career or workplace should be identified and managed.

---

anatomē's
WORKPLACE ANXIETY ASSESSMENT

If you stress beyond acceptable levels and it relates to aspects of your work, make sure you identify it. Here are some questions worth answering:

1 Do you struggle to switch off after a workday?

2 Is your relationship with your colleagues tense?

3 Do you worry about making mistakes, keeping paper trails, or being misinterpreted when presenting or communicating at work?

4 Does your job feel highly unsafe?

5 Do you strongly disagree with the values of your workplace?

6 Are you afraid of failure to the point of being frozen and not knowing how to conduct business?

While the above situations may arise at some point, an ongoing relationship with work in which these feelings prevail is likely to harm your health and wellness.

Assessing it may indicate it's time for a career or job change. You may also decide to manage these feelings while maintaining your current job. Either way, we recommend the following steps to help you manage your work anxiety and keep it from taking over other aspects of your life.

STEPS FOR WELLBEING IN THE WORKPLACE

1 Read this out loud: 'A job is just a job'

While it may be a source of income, affirmation and even an extension of who you are, separating your work from your other life facets will help you relativize the importance of it, relieving some of the anxiety caused by your efforts to keep or excel at it.

2 Switch off the overtime

Whether you own a business or work as an employee, if working extra hours every day is an expectation, there is something wrong. And it can be either with you or with your job. Strict management of your work time and a firm decision to say no to overtime will release time for your personal endeavours and pleasures, automatically reducing the weight of work in your lifestyle. Of course, we all put in some extra effort when a big pitch or a deadline is coming up. But anything beyond that momentary peak is unhealthy and should be stopped. Communicate your decision or phase it out by gradually reducing your hours. If you work from home, turn your computer off at the right time: when your work is done or when your manageable work hours are completed. It's important to have a set limit, based on your role and responsibilities, that ensure your workload and time employed are sustainable – medium and long term.

3 Keep a separate work phone

If you have that second phone – the one with a different cover – which you use to take work calls and receive emails, great! Make sure it's turned off at any unreasonable hour (depending on your job). Mobile work devices are proven efficiency facilitators. But they can generate stress if you don't know when to switch them off. If you manage work and personal lives from the same phone, consider taking a second device.

4 Distinguish friends from colleagues

This advice may seem harsh, but we need to address it. That work colleague with whom you get a weekly drink to catch up on the office gossip may be harming your mental wellbeing without anyone noticing. Whether the conversation is light-hearted, humorous or serious, exchanging unofficial work information and, consequently, opinions and speculations about it, will likely help trigger your anxiety. Cutting back on workplace friendships may mean you'll be less in the know about the office gossip but, in this case, ignorance is bliss. The more you know about rumours from your workplace, the more likely you are to internalize it, project or transfer the anxiety it will generate.

5 Take lunch breaks

A well-managed workday should always include an entire hour to unwind in the middle of the day. Take this time to go for a walk, have lunch on your own or even call someone from outside the office. This small gesture will help you put anything stressful that may have happened in the morning in perspective – and establish a clear mind for the afternoon ahead of you.

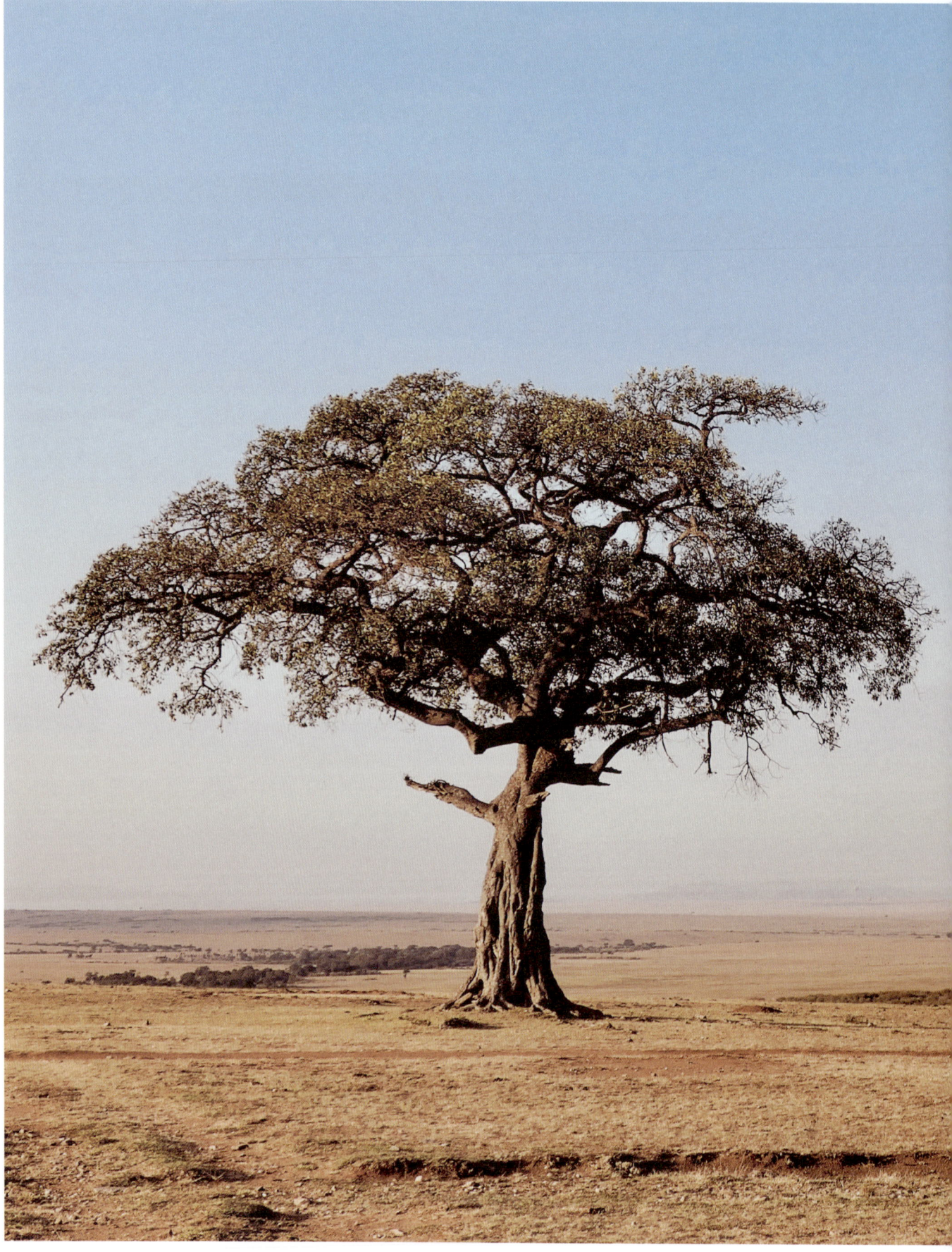

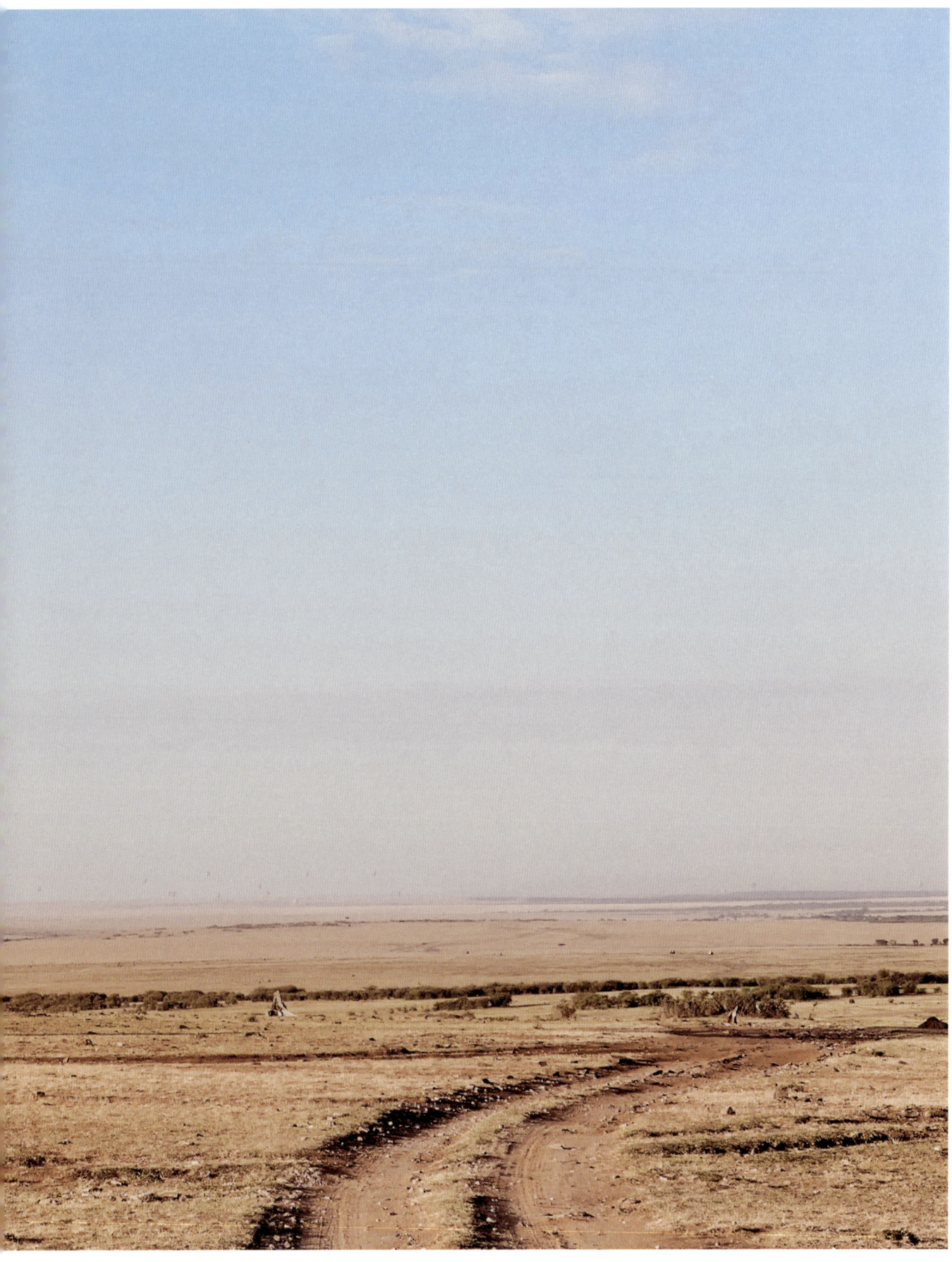

3 SCREEN TIME

Six hours, 58 minutes: the time people globally spend in front of screens every day. That makes up for 27 per cent of our day. If you remove sleeping time (8 hours, if you're being good), you have 41 per cent.

Your screen time may be even higher if you have an intense desktop workday, a Netflix binge in the evening and a lot of phone time in between. While being connected is a part of modern life, living in front of the screen affects our wellbeing – psychologically and physically.

You're probably reading this chapter thinking you'll have to ignore the recommendations listed, since there is no way you can reduce your screen time. Don't give up just yet. Understanding the impact of screens and then managing your relationship with them – even if just to gain a mere 15 minutes on your first attempt – will pay off.

Let's divide screen overtime impact into two types: physical and psychological. We will assess them separately and then combine our recommendations to help you achieve mind and body improvements as you manage this particular aspect of your life.

PHYSICAL
▪ Sedentarism
Screen time is still-body time, in most cases (if you walk while texting, then we have a different danger to address, maybe in another book). We use our desktops, phones, tablets, TVs and video games while sitting or lying still. While we can try to find a comfortable position to do it, these activities correspond to sedentary time, when we're not exercising.

Sedentarism leads to a reduction in calories used, accumulation of fat in the body, and, ultimately, obesity and its consequences, putting us at higher risk of developing high blood pressure, type 2 diabetes and increased levels of bad cholesterol (LDL).

▪ Chronic body pain
We're mainly talking neck and back – and this is serious. Screen time – each screen with its specific factors – can lead to incorrect posture and hence to chronic pain.

Think about that bent neck while you're using your phone. An incorrect posture you can't shake off when you're in front of your laptop. While you can strive for the best possible posture to look at your screen, the risk of strain on your body from a prolonged time in a repeated unnatural position remains.

PSYCHOLOGICAL
▪ Sleep problems
We will get to it in more detail, but sleep is highly affected by the lights emitted by screens. You may not notice it, but looking at the bright lights emitted by your electronic devices is telling your brain it's bright daytime, interfering with your sleep cycle.

DEPRESSION AND ANXIETY
The time spent in front of a screen is time you're not spending connecting with the world around you. Depending on the content you're looking at – from passive-aggressive work emails to frantic reels to creepy series to rude texts – you're likely overstimulated, which can cause mental fatigue, stress, anxiety and depression.

anatomē's
GUIDE TO MANAGING YOUR SCREEN TIME

The only way to reduce the impact of screens on your wellbeing is to manage your screen time.

Here are some guidelines: pick and choose the ones that suit you.

Know your screen time stats
Knowledge is half the battle here. Work out how many of your work hours are spent in front of the screen. You may want to work on an average if your days aren't always the same. And work out how many episodes of your favourite series you watch every night. Do the same for video games, tablets, online shopping and any other type of screen time.

Set up a goal and decide where you'll cut off
If you choose to reduce your overall screen time by 10 per cent, for example, work out this time in minutes. You'll then decide on what to cut off. If you can't possibly reduce your work email time, try declining a meeting of minor importance, deleting an app that's consuming too much time, or even cutting back on one episode of your favourite show a week.

Your smartphone has digital wellbeing tools that calculate your screen time, classifying it to help you identify excesses.

Find an off-screen activity
During an hour or more daily, engage in an activity that doesn't involve screen time. It can be your gym time, a run, cooking, reading or anything you find enjoyable. This time in your day should be kept religiously and with no interruptions. Put your phone away, close your laptop and turn the TV off. Remember how you felt during this time off-screen. If your time was peaceful, think about ways to increase it. If you feel anxious and tempted to reach for the nearest screen, keep trying: it gets better.

Take short breaks
During prolonged screen-focused activities, take short breaks. It can be a pause for refreshments, a short walk around the block or even a stretch away from the desk. A 5-minute break from the screen every hour or so will improve your productivity and keep you connected with the world around you, protecting your mental health and physical wellbeing from the dangers of screen time.

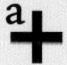

4 UNBALANCED DIET

Diet isn't just a matter of fuelling the body. It's also how we obtain all the additives that allow it to perform chemical reactions responsible for our living. Aside from the oxygen we breathe, everything that feeds our bodies comes from our diet.

And the choices we make will define how the body will perform – including muscles, mind and every function performed by each organ.

We all know we need to have a balanced diet, and there is enough literature available for you to address it. Therefore, to maintain our focus on practices and awareness, we will look at the habits that promote 'bad eating' in modern living and give you a few ideas to manage your food and drink consumption to improve your wellbeing.

Forget calorie intake for now. Have the number of your recommended calorie count based on your gender, weight, height, lifestyle and health aspects. If you're not sure, find out with a specialist. We will focus on habits and how you can change them to improve your routine without prescribing a complete regime, which is a job for a registered nutritionist or a physician.

anatomē's
LIST OF DIET VILLAINS

Here is a short list of bad eating habits and some recommendations for how to change them.

Overeating
Recent studies have revealed that, for the first time in human history, the number of individuals overeating is higher than those not eating enough (hunger). Sadly, both indexes continue to rise. While obesity is the most well-known manifestation of overeating, an increasing number of individuals ingest more calories than recommended.

Lack of dietary quality
Calories aren't just calories. The nutritional value and the level of processing involved in preparing the food we consume have the same weight in a balanced diet. For commodity, economy or habit, we resort to packaged meals, snacks, fast food and takeaways, at times spending long periods relying on them to satisfy our hunger. It's not only about 'empty calories', but also calories filled with badness (think unhealthy fats, added sugars and sodium).

Snacking
Regular meals with breaks during which our bodies digest the food allow for the correct absorption of nutrients, regulate insulin and blood sugar and even help control our appetite. Snacking not only throws off our digestive rhythm but it also means we may be adding poor choices to the menu, as snacks are often nutrient-poor.

Fast eating
It happens to many of us. We become accustomed to squeezing meals between meetings, not taking the time to chew and swallow our food correctly. Fast eating, aside from being frowned upon for etiquette and increasing chances of choking and hiccups, can be highly damaging to our bodies.

Fast eating can cause erosive gastritis – caused by the strain on the internal lining of the stomach – and metabolic syndrome, also known as insulin resistance, which is likely to increase the risk of type 2 diabetes, heart disease and stroke.

Eating too fast also leads to overeating, not allowing time for ghrelin, the hormone that tells us we are hungry, to reach the brain and tell it 'we're satisfied'.

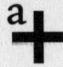

anatomē's
STEPS FOR A BALANCED DIET

A diet of nutritionally rich, whole and unprocessed foods promotes fewer mood swings, better sleep and improved focus, and even helps fight anxiety and depression.

With the risk of boring you with information you've already read, here are some of our favourite ways to enjoy a balanced diet.

Log your food intake
We recommend downloading an app and logging everything you eat and drink in one day. Following the principle of 'knowing is half the battle', this measure will help you understand the pros and cons of your food, help keep track of your nutrition and plan necessary changes that fit within your lifestyle.

Plan at least one of your daily meals
If you don't have complete control of where and when you'll get a chance to eat, selecting one meal and changing it into a nutritionally rich, sensible dish is a way of improving your overall dietary intake. Make sure you add plenty of protein and fibre to this meal, which will help control hunger throughout the day.

Identify emotional or stress eating
More common than we'd like to admit, emotional eating is another cause of poor diet. It refers to anything not ingested for pleasure or as fuel: feeding boredom, anger, stress and even lack of sleep. When we're out of balance, some resort to food to numb their emotions. If this rings a bell, a simple awareness of these moments can help you to fight them.

Eat before going food shopping
Shopping on an empty stomach is a route to bad decision-making. Whether shopping online or physically, do it after a well-balanced meal. You'll remove emotional influence and keep momentary cravings from informing your weekly shop. When your home has no nutritionally poor snacks, you're less likely to succumb to them.

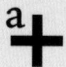

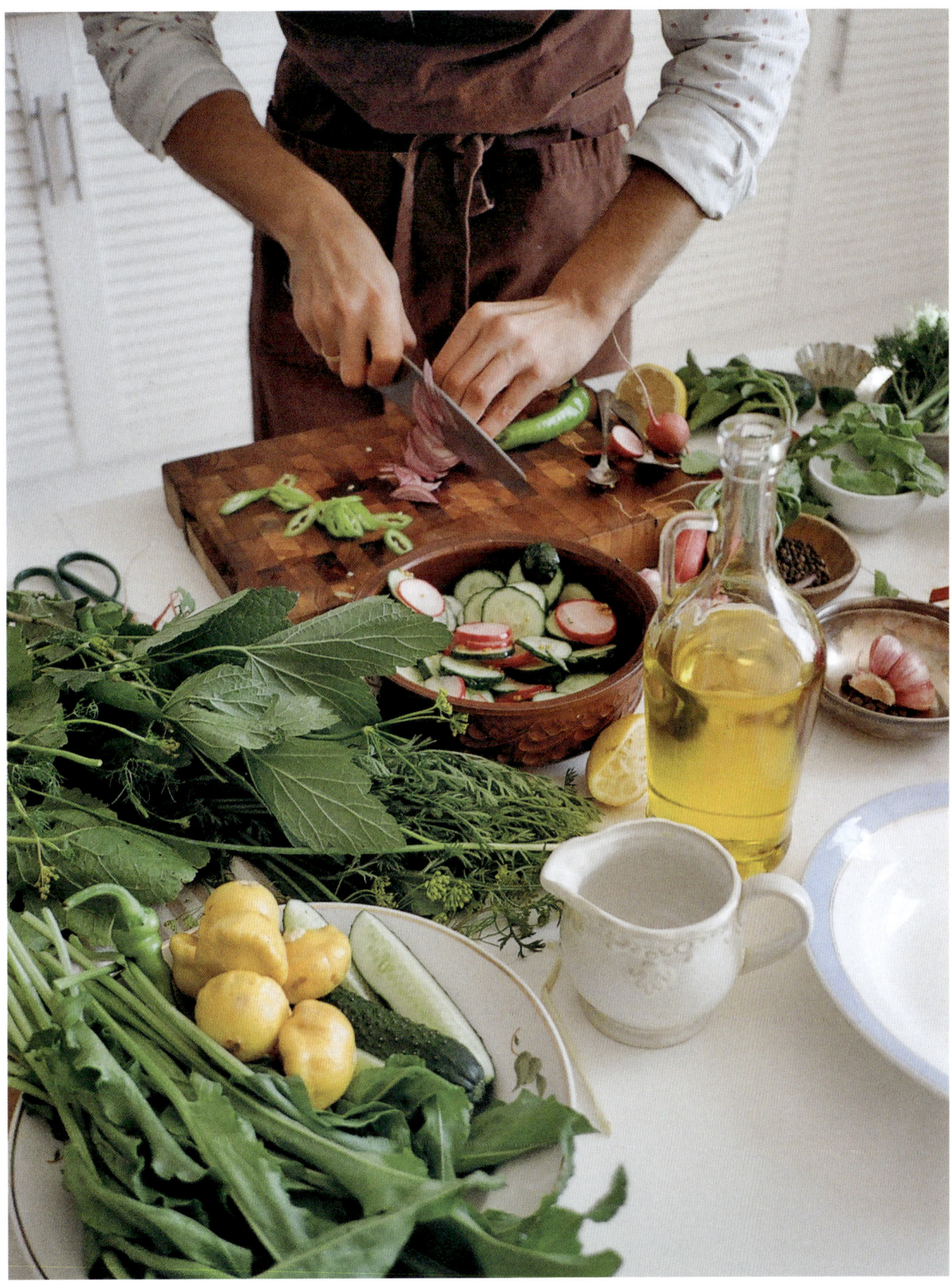

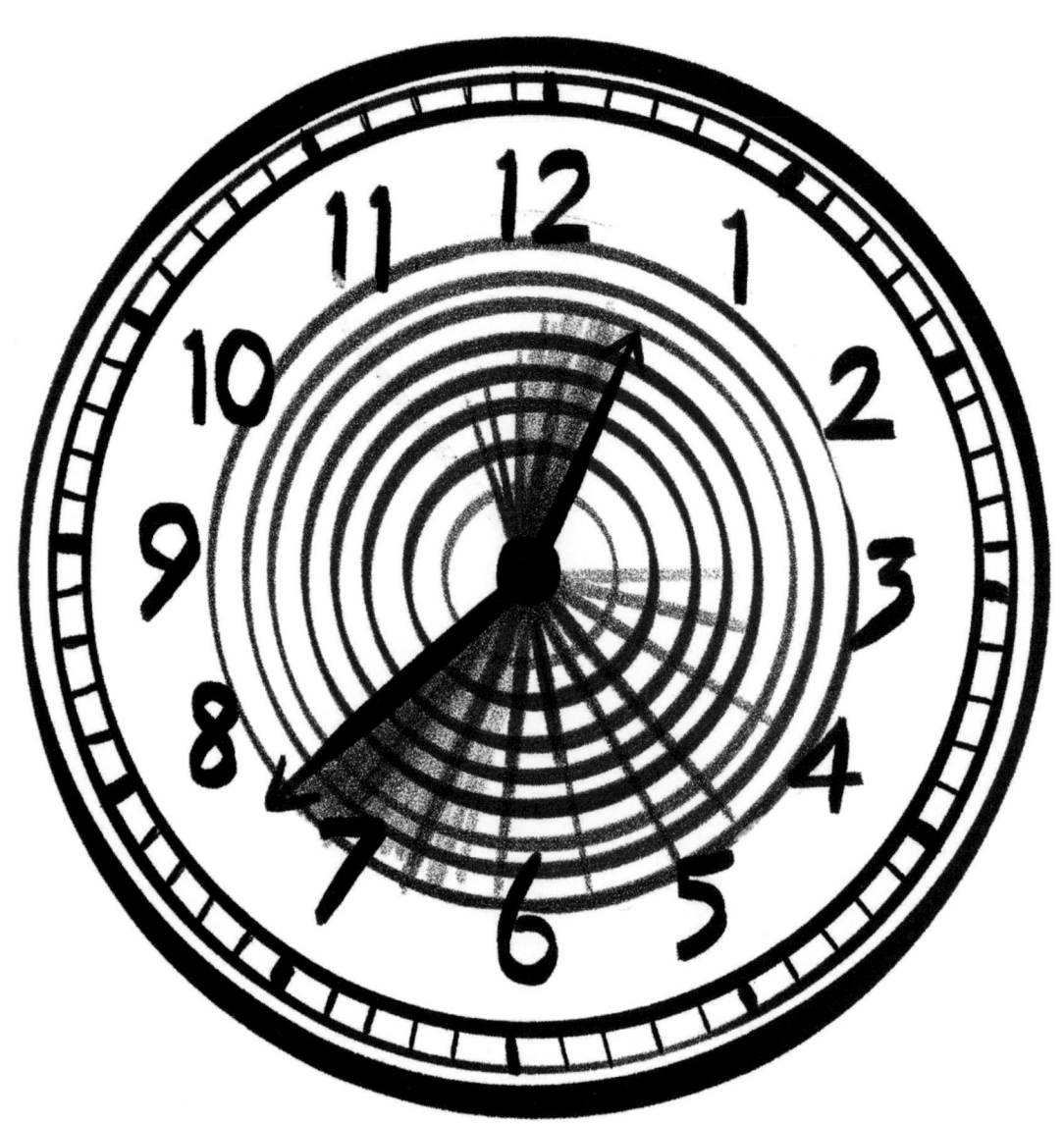

5 TIME (OR LACK THEREOF)

Before discussing time management and the effects of 'having no time' on our wellbeing, let's establish that the concept of time is relative. Under no circumstances should we compare our time and use of it with someone else's. Our daily load of activities, thoughts and approach to them are individual, non-transferable and incomparable.

Whether consciously or not, our days always start with a thought: what do I need to do today? Modern society glorifies 'being busy', imposing it on children from an early age, shaming teenagers for their hormonal idleness and dividing adults into 'hard workers' and 'slackers'.

'I'm so busy' is modern jargon used to set the tone at work, justify our social absence and create a sense of earnestness. But a deeper quality analysis of our busyness may indicate that we're accumulating activities but performing at a quality level below our capacities, while harming our mental health and wellbeing.

Being busy becomes dangerous when it affects your ability to look after yourself, dedicate time to collect your thoughts and recharge after a period of intense performance. Excessive busyness can lead to burnout, performance issues, anxiety and depression, along with all the physical health risks these states cause.

So, before you spell out 'I'm so busy' under your breath, in your head or to someone else, let's focus on a few steps to make busyness productive, qualitative and mentally safe. Wouldn't it be a treat to replace this jargon with something more unique and engaging?

Time management is not just an HR term. And it doesn't just apply to work. In your 16 waking hours (assuming you managed to get your 8-hour sleep), you must have time to complete your daily tasks with quality, leaving a percentage of this time for self-care, reflection and enjoyable activities. And that is non-negotiable. If you can't find time to exercise, eat a healthy meal or even watch a series to help you unwind, you're not managing your time correctly, overcommitting or self-sabotaging.

Based on conversations with our customers and community members, we created anatomē's short guide for time management. It applies to work, social life and families. Use it wherever it applies in your life.

1 Write the list, with a twist

We wouldn't simply tell you to write a to-do list. We have a more sophisticated approach to it. While the list, or as we also say journal, helps you go through your tasks in an orderly manner by relieving some of the stress of disorganized information floating in your brain, a strict list can backfire by imposing efficiency, forcing you to speed up or extend your efforts to complete tasks.

The anatomē list is more comprehensive. Take the time to write your to-do list. Then go back, task by task, and think about a shortcut, the possibility of pushing the deadline or delegating. Firmly relativize and find ways of turning this list into a strategic document that helps you govern your life. It can present solutions as simple as replacing stopping by the supermarket with ordering online or making a note next to 'prepare presentation': get an assistant to do it.

2 Identify and interrupt guilt trips

We're all on our own journeys. And they're not easy. While compassion, friendship and caring for others should be part of our lives, giving too much time away for others – this includes family and close friends – will likely drain your energy and disposition, consume your time and affect your ability to look after yourself and anyone else.

You don't need to answer the phone every time someone calls, text messages can wait and declining invitations to preserve your time is utterly acceptable.

If you're spending a large percentage of your time – free or allocated – catering to others' needs, establish boundaries. Saying 'No' and explaining the situation can be uncomfortable at first, but is guaranteed to benefit you in the long run.

3 Allocate me time and stick with it

If you treat your free time as anyone's time, others will too. The fact that you're not working or don't have a social commitment at a given moment doesn't mean the time is up for grabs. Normalize establishing that you're busy with yourself, create fake meetings on your work calendar to take an hour back and say no, explaining a given time is reserved for self-care. Once the initial awkwardness is out of the way, you'll notice your other activities will fall into place, people will adapt to your rhythm and you'll enjoy the benefits of having time in the week reserved for you.

4 Take the time for the small gestures

A characteristic of busyness is not taking the time for smaller tasks. Taking an extra 10 minutes to pack your kids' lunch, making a homemade sandwich, ironing your favourite shirt, or spending another 5 minutes on your beauty practice or listening to a song before you get on a call will fill your day with moments of awareness and presence, helping you relativize the importance of your tasks, and establishing a more serene approach to 'just doing it'.

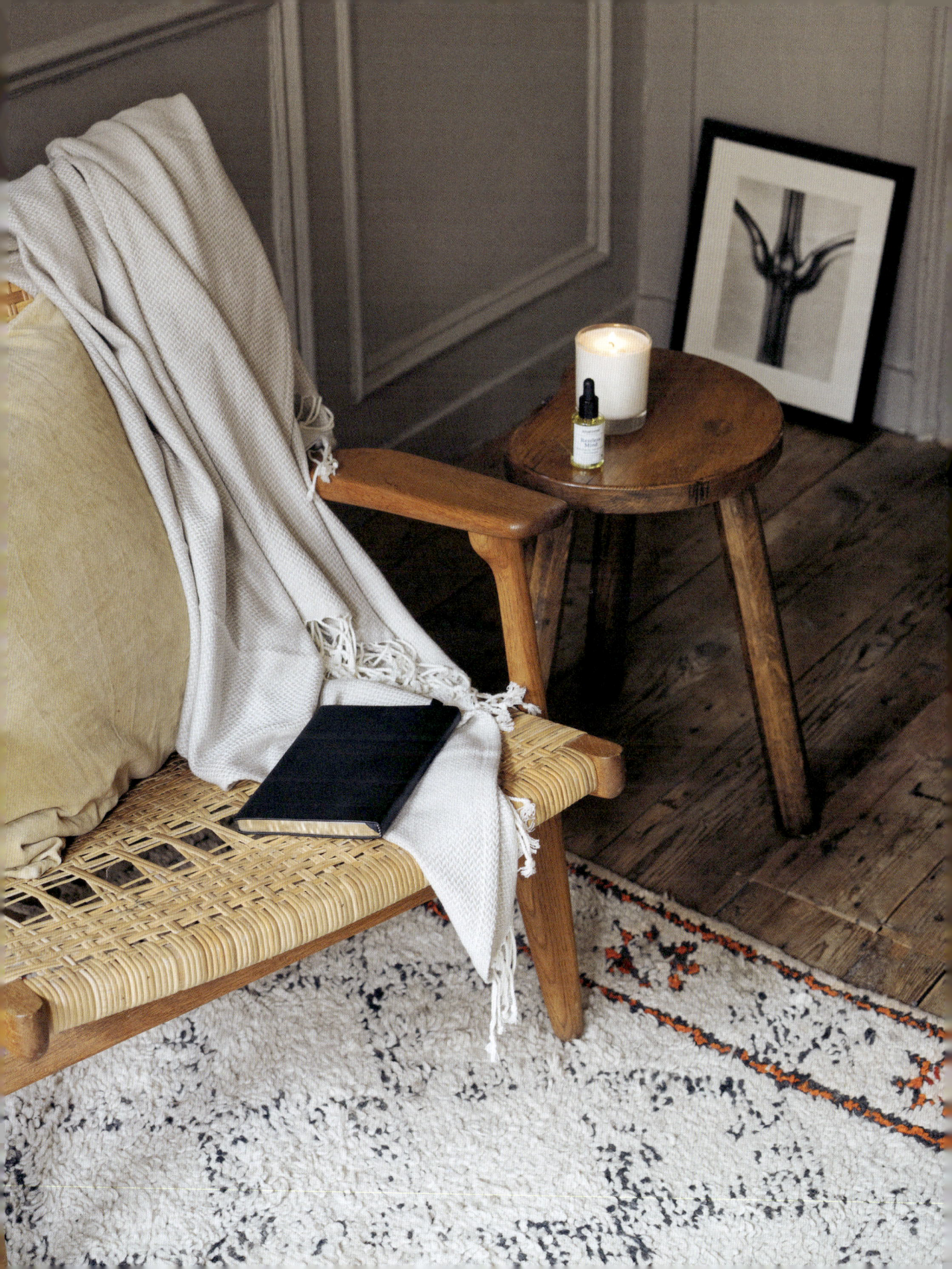

WEL

PRA

LBEING

CTICES

WHAT ARE WELLBEING PRACTICES?

Your botanical formulations will work to help you feel better.
But they work as a part of a regime.

At anatomē, we call them practices. They are guidelines we share with our communities to help them make the most of their formulations. When we created them, the idea was to bring positive exercises, postures and mindfulness exercises together with the gestures of utilizing the formulas, ultimately converting empty or 'wasted' time into self-care, feel-better moments.

On average, we spend 2½ hours a day on social media – probably the most mindless activity in our day. We believe that converting a fraction of this time into practice time will promote a significant positive change in how you feel.

A wellbeing practice isn't a task like a personal training session. It's also not a prescriptive ritual to follow to a T. A wellbeing practice is easy to repeat, gives us a little break from all the other activities in the day, and converts mindless time into a precious few minutes that transform our minds and, with time, our bodies.

Your practices must work for you, fit (almost) seamlessly into your routine and be a pleasure, never a chore. You should look forward to your wellbeing practices and never dread them.

A wellbeing practice is more than simply using your oils, candles and skincare. The idea is to promote a wellbeing system in which your body welcomes the benefits of the scents but also promotes their healing functions, slows down and offers a feel-good effect.

These are suggestions and can be tailored and adapted as you wish. The following steps relate to any practice and can also be applied to everyday activities.

COMMIT TO A TIME

Whichever practice you adopt will require time. You'll need to make a few minutes, preferably at the same time every day, and stick to it.

Time commitment and discipline are easy to recommend. In the age of FoMO (see page 118) and overbooked individuals and families, however, it can be the biggest challenge between ourselves and our self-care.

Many anatomē community members have reported on their journeys to create their practices. A great majority have mentioned their fight against external stimuli to make time for their self-care moments. For many, this 'practice' felt superfluous, selfish and disposable – no matter how aware they were of how beneficial the practices were.

- Choose a convenient time for your practice.
- If necessary, create a reminder on your phone.
- Let others know you are not available during this time (including your children, partner, colleagues and friends).
- Decline appointments that clash with your practice time.
- Stay away from your phone during your practice.
- Remind yourself of the importance of this time for your wellbeing.

Start small. If you feel comfortable committing to 5 minutes, that's your practice time. You can increase it as you feel ready. You can even find another time if your circumstances change.

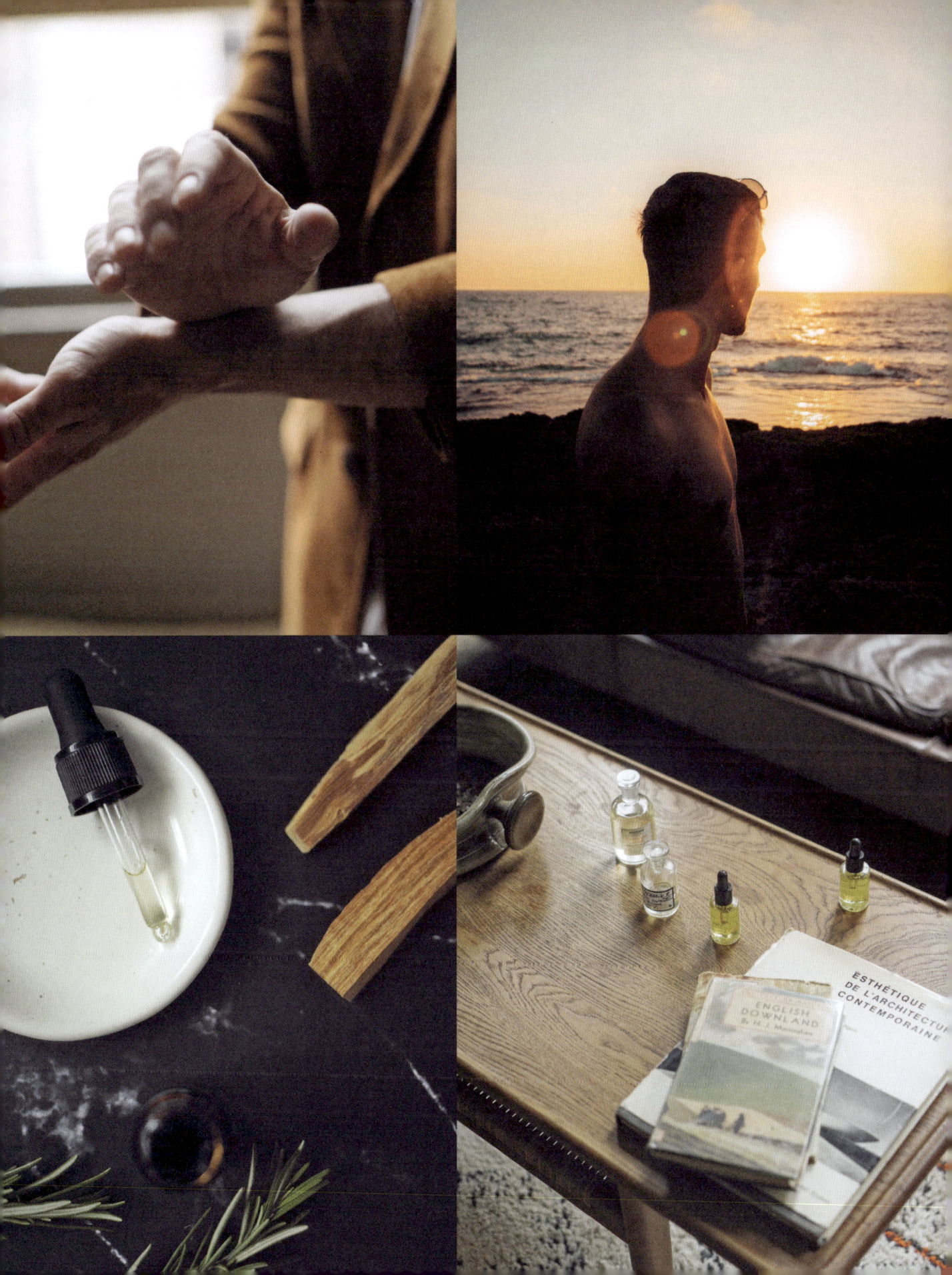

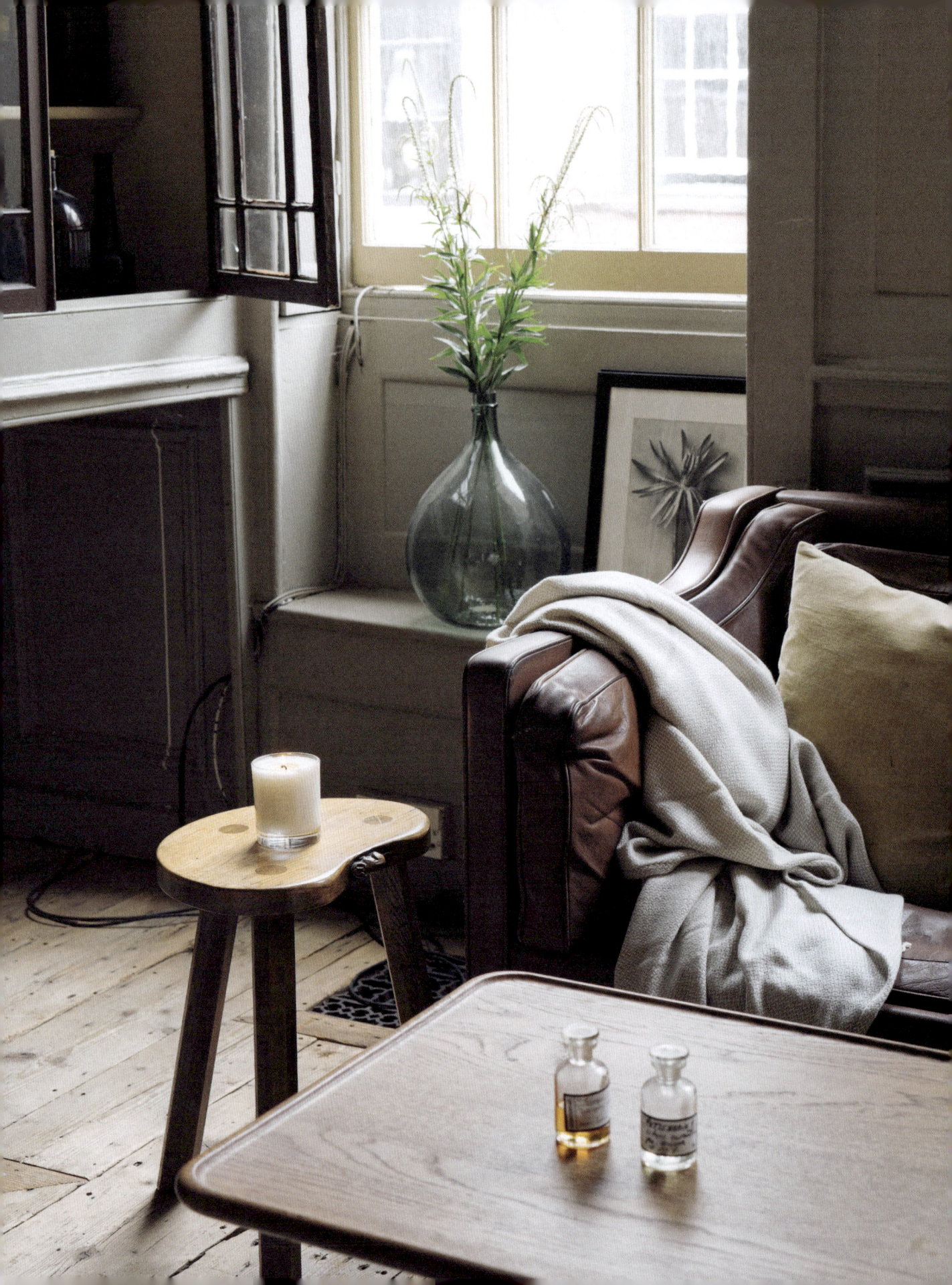

CURATE YOUR SPACE

The COVID-19 pandemic made us all more focused on our living spaces. We learned DIY skills, paid attention to details of our homes we hadn't noticed before and developed a taste – and a need – to feel more comfortable in our homes.

Interior design can focus on curation, collection and artistic expression – and an impressive, sophisticated home can be incredibly uplifting. But joyful living happens in spaces where we can be ourselves. Put our feet up, be creative and shelter from the world.

In your space, it doesn't matter if you're lying on a mid-century leather sofa staring at contemporary artwork bought at Miami Basel, resting your cocktail on a travertine side table. It's about feeling peaceful, having your favourite belongings near you and being sure you can do no wrong while there.

While you won't necessarily be in the same place every day, having a place in your home or your workspace where you feel safe and serene will help you establish your practice. The familiarity – and sheer repetition of place – will help your mind establish a habit.

An ideal space is a place where you exist with no compromise. You want to make sure your children's toys aren't lying on the floor and that your mother-in-law's picture isn't staring at you.

This place can be your bathroom if your practice is skincare or a bath. If you have a bedtime practice, your bedroom will be the place for it. But, in theory, a wellbeing practice can take place anywhere: garden, kitchen, living room or even at your desk.

If you're lucky enough to have such a place, decorate it with objects, colours and textures that reflect you. While we recommend avoiding clutter, there's nothing wrong with a few trinkets that bring a smile to your face.

Have all the items you need for your practice to hand, organized and ready to use.

Strictly no screens allowed. That includes phones, computers, tablets and TVs. You also want to remove to-do lists, bills and anything that reminds you of the outside world and its challenges.

Adjust the lighting to serve your purpose. You want darkness to help you relax and unwind, but if you're working on your skin, you will need better lighting to help your practice.

If your space is a silent place, once again, you're lucky. If not, the tips on the following pages will help you zone out anything from traffic noises to loud children. You can play music or sounds that help your mind focus on the moment.

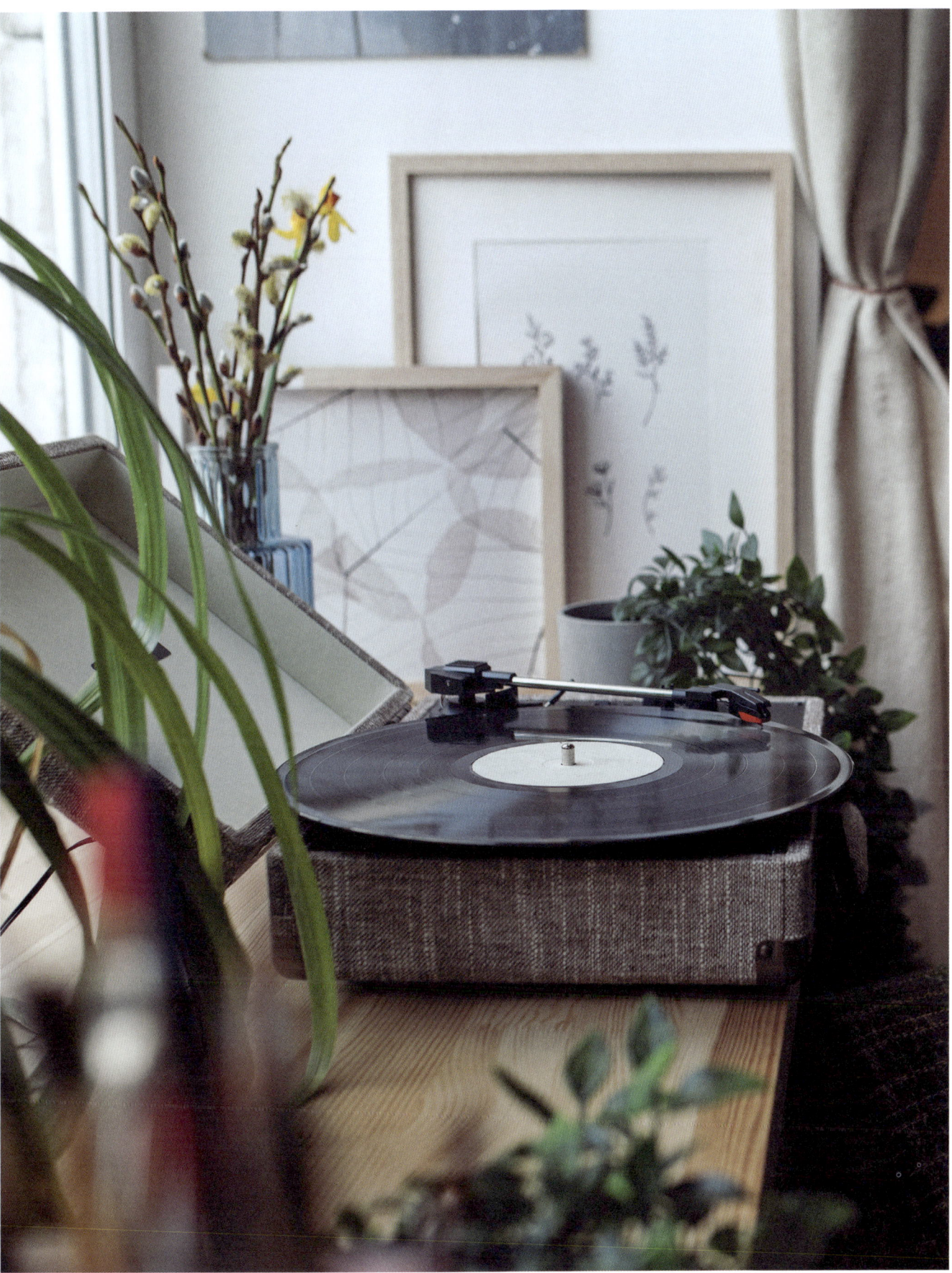

MIND THE BODY

You've probably heard from someone that you need to work on your posture. You've probably heard it from someone who also needs to work on theirs.

We will not do it yet again. For your daily practice, we recommend that you think about your body. Try to identify the sensation in each part of the body. Find tension, mild pains, pressure and anything that may feel uncomfortable. Intuitively, try to adjust your body to ease these minor discomforts.

Need something a little more prescriptive to get started? Here is some general posture advice:

If you're sitting down, your feet should rest flat on the floor. Distribute your weight evenly on your hips. Keep your back straight. Shoulders back, relaxed, keeping your ears aligned with your collarbones.

If you stand during your practice, bend your knees slightly so they're not 'locked', protecting your joints.

Remember that better posture can feel awkward at first. Many of us are conditioned to hunch, slouch and twist throughout the day. Addressing your posture daily for a few minutes will likely help you think about it more frequently. Embrace this possibility.

TAKE A FEW DEEP BREATHS

When people tell you to take a deep breath, even though they may just be giving generic advice – something they repeat because it sounds appropriate – it works when you are feeling overwhelmed, stressed or about to make an impulsive decision.

Politeness aside, breathing exercises are scientifically proven to help you focus and relax. The technique below works through both neurobiological and psychological mechanisms. And it's simple to follow:

Inhale slowly through your nose, completely filling your lungs with air. Hold your breath for a second. Exhale at the same pace until you've emptied your lungs. Repeat a few times.

The goal is to align the pace of your breath with that of your heart rate, ultimately stabilizing your heartbeat. It will then increase the activity of the vagus nerve, part of our parasympathetic nervous system, which controls many of our organs.

Stimulating the vagus nerve will help your body calm down. If increased, your heart rate will slow down, your blood pressure will decrease and your muscles will naturally relax.

Ultimately, the same nerve will inform the brain of the slower overall rhythm of the body. The brain will adjust to it, producing satisfying feelings of peacefulness.

SLEEP PRACTICE

If your sleeplessness is the result of a stressful modern lifestyle, then you can start with a sleep practice. Just to note, before assessing your sleep, make sure you've already eliminated all clinical conditions that could be causing insomnia. You must treat any medical condition first, even if you adopt a sleep practice to support any treatment.

1 Pre-sleep detox. Give your body time to clear from sleep-harming substances and stimuli. Here's how far before bedtime you need to clear from each of them:

- **Alcohol**: 2 hours
- **Caffeine**: 6 hours
- **Screens**: 1 hour
- **Social media**: 2 hours
- **Emails**: 2 hours
- **Smoking**: 1 hour
- **Exercise**: 1 hour
- **Food**: 2 hours
- **Loud music and noise**: 1 hour

2 Set up a sleep time and stick to it. It's not an easy task, and it may require some anti-social decisions, such as declining invites. That said, you may discover the benefits of leaving a party when it's at its peak, limiting your presence and making more of reduced hours of social interaction. Whatever you do, get to bed at the same time every night. It pays off.

3 Establish a quiet, relaxing bedtime routine. For example, drink a cup of caffeine-free tea, take a warm shower or listen to soft music. Avoid prolonged use of electronic devices with a screen, such as laptops, smartphones and ebooks before bed.

4 Relax your body. Gentle yoga or progressive muscle relaxation can ease tension and help tight muscles relax.

5 Make your bedroom conducive to sleep. Keep light, noise and temperature at comfortable levels that won't disturb your rest. Don't engage in activities other than sleeping or having sex in your bedroom. This will help your body know this room is for sleeping (and sex).

6 Put clocks in your bedroom out of sight. We've all been there: the vicious cycle of not sleeping and then feeling even more restless as you watch the time and calculate how many hours you'll get before waking up. Clock-watching causes stress and makes it harder to go back to sleep if you wake up during the night.

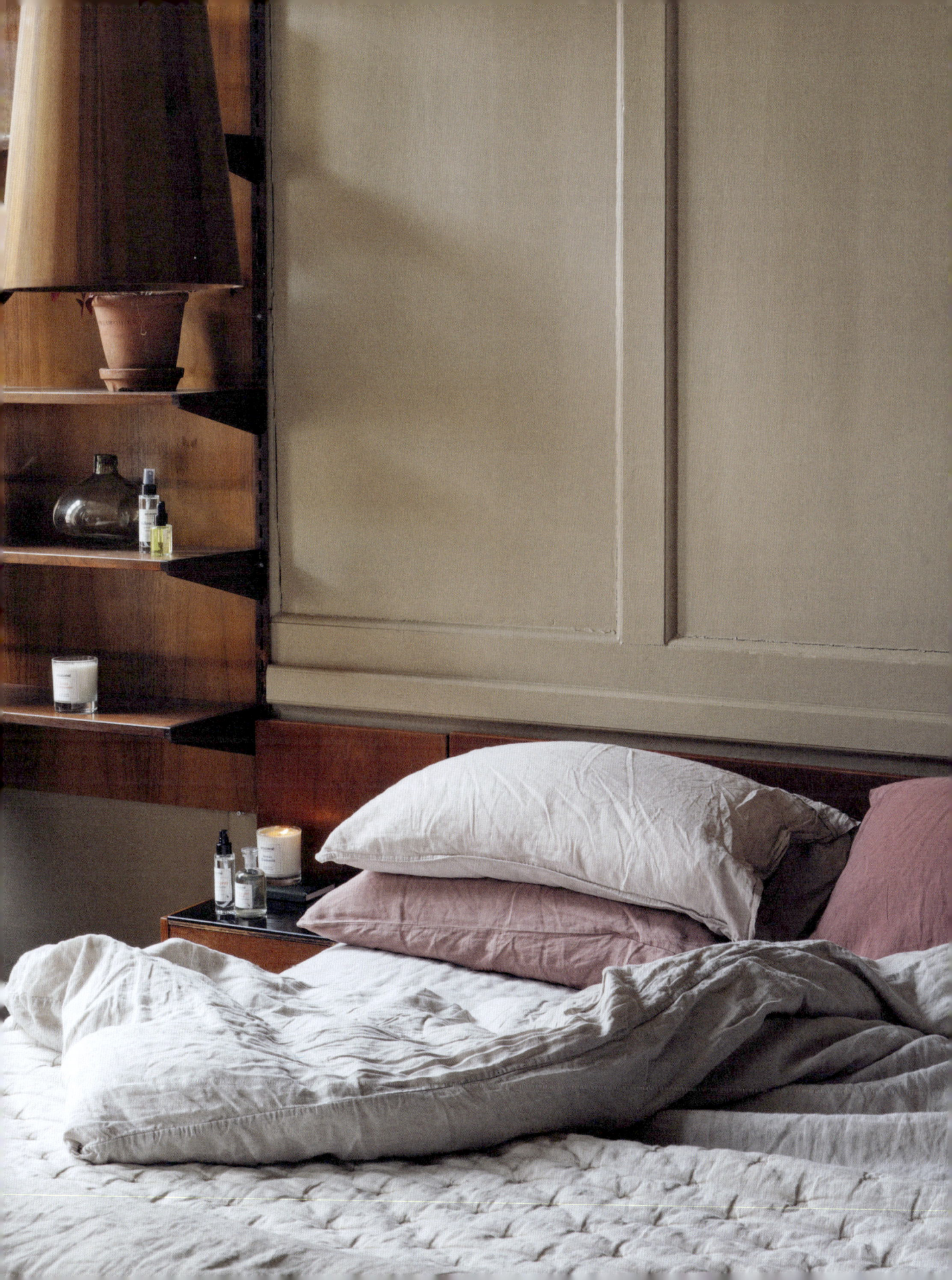

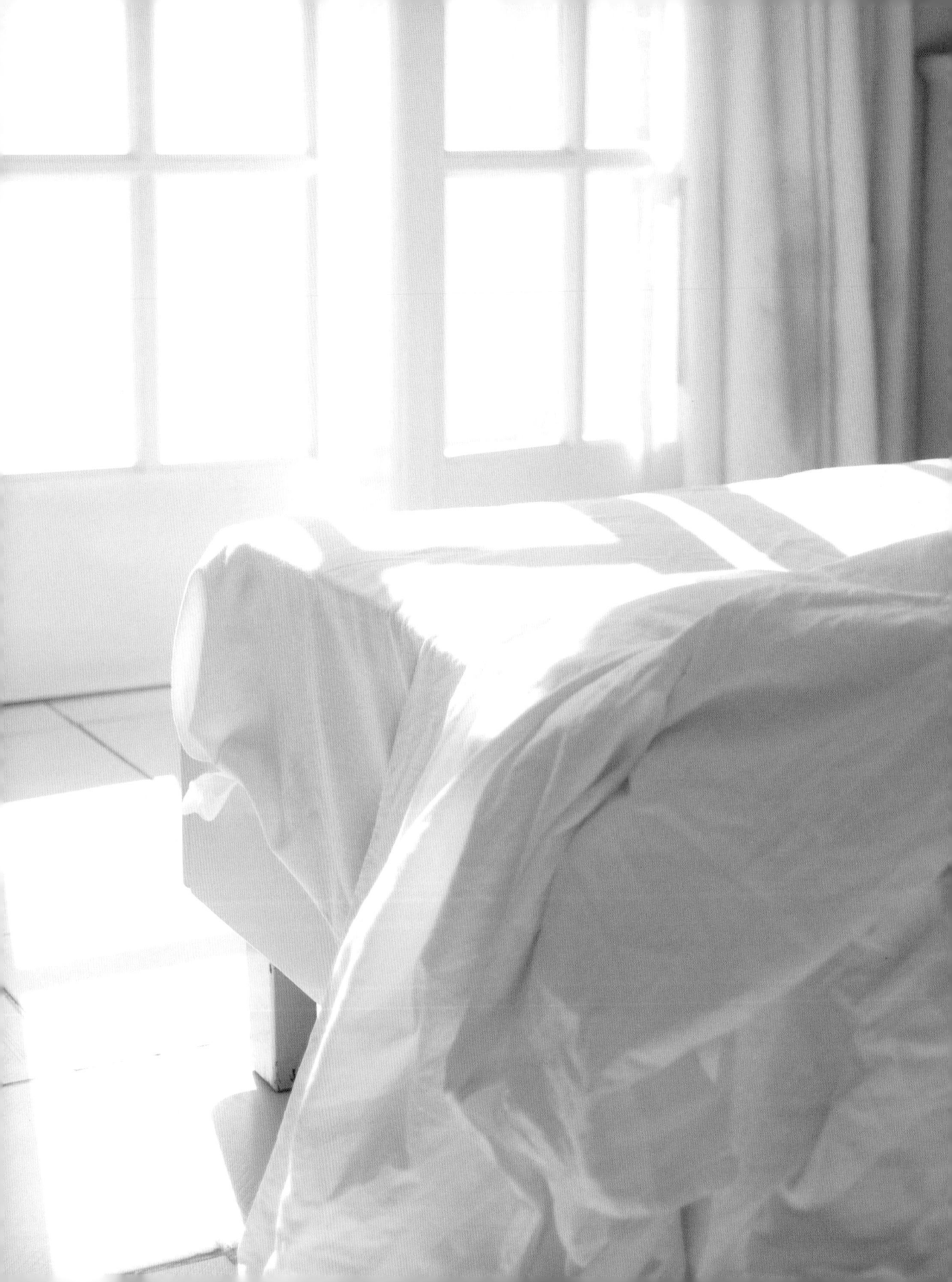

7 **Get regular exercise, but not before bedtime.** You will need to rethink late workouts or that night run. Even though exercise is an excellent way of reducing stress, it does increase your heart rate and awakens the body.

8 **Go to bed only when you're sleepy.** If you aren't sleepy by bedtime, find an activity that helps your brain unwind. Make it a screen-free activity, such as knitting, reading or even meditating.

9 **Wake up at the same time every day.** The discipline of sleep can be taught. Your body will respond to a structured sleep routine, so even on weekends, maintain a consistent wake-up time (we know: this one may bite). If you experience increased awake time at night, resist the urge to sleep in.

10 **Avoid daytime napping.** Napping can throw off your sleep cycle. Even 1 hour of sleep during the day may tell your body that sleep is done and dusted. Resist the urge to nap during the day, especially if it's not something you can enjoy daily.

11 **If you wake up and can't fall back to sleep within 20 minutes or so, get out of bed.** By doing so, you'll be telling your body it gets to start over. Read, make yourself a non-caffeinated tea, drink some water (not much, to avoid waking up to use the loo), and repeat your entire bedtime routine when you feel ready.

THE BENEFITS OF DEEP BREATHING BEFORE BED

After a day of study, work or any busyness, our brains can get into overthinking mode. That, aligned with worries about the coming day and the inevitable counting of sleep hours lost, come together to keep us wide awake.

An American psychology study in Massachusetts showed that deep breathing, aligned with mindfulness, helps calm the nervous system, silence those thoughts and promote better, restful sleep.

Breathing practices can be challenging for stubborn minds – but sticking with them will pay off. Understanding the science behind these techniques will convince you to try harder than you have previously.

Practising breathing before bed slows the heart rate and tells our brains it's time to relax and unwind. Once the brain is relaxed and sleepy, the rest of the body naturally follows suit.

Deep breathing before bed produces a life-changing mindfulness effect, forcing the brain to focus on controlling breathing rather than on distractions in our minds. By suppressing the noise in the brain, we can reach the so-wanted relaxed state faster and fall asleep in less time.

Breathing techniques to help promote sleep vary. You may have learned something different from what you'll see opposite. Stick with one and repeat it persistently. The goal is the same – and so are the results.

anatomē's
GUIDE TO ABDOMINAL BREATHING

Abdominal or belly breathing – technically known as diaphragmatic breathing – encourages deep breathing from the stomach rather than the chest. Here's how to do it:

1 Sit or lie down in a comfortable place. Close your eyes.
2 Place one hand on your chest and one on your stomach. As you breathe, the lower hand should move. The top hand remains stationary or only moves when the bottom hand moves.
3 Breathe through your nose for about 4 seconds and feel your stomach expand. (You may feel a slight strain during the first few breaths.)
4 Hold your breath for 2 seconds.
5 Exhale slowly and evenly through your mouth for about 6 seconds. The mouth should be relaxed.
6 Repeat for 5–15 minutes.

anatomē's
GUIDE TO 4-7-8 BREATHING TECHNIQUE

During this exercise, place the tip of your tongue against the edge of the tissue behind your upper front teeth while exhaling through your mouth around your tongue. Then follow these steps:

1 Exhale completely through your mouth and make a hissing sound. With your mouth closed, breathe in slowly through your nose and mentally count to four.
2 Then hold your breath and count to seven.
3 Exhaling through your mouth, make a whooshing sound and count to eight.
4 Repeat three times, for a total of four breathing cycles. Focus on maintaining a 4-count, 7-count and 8-count ratio: that is more important than the time spent in each phase.

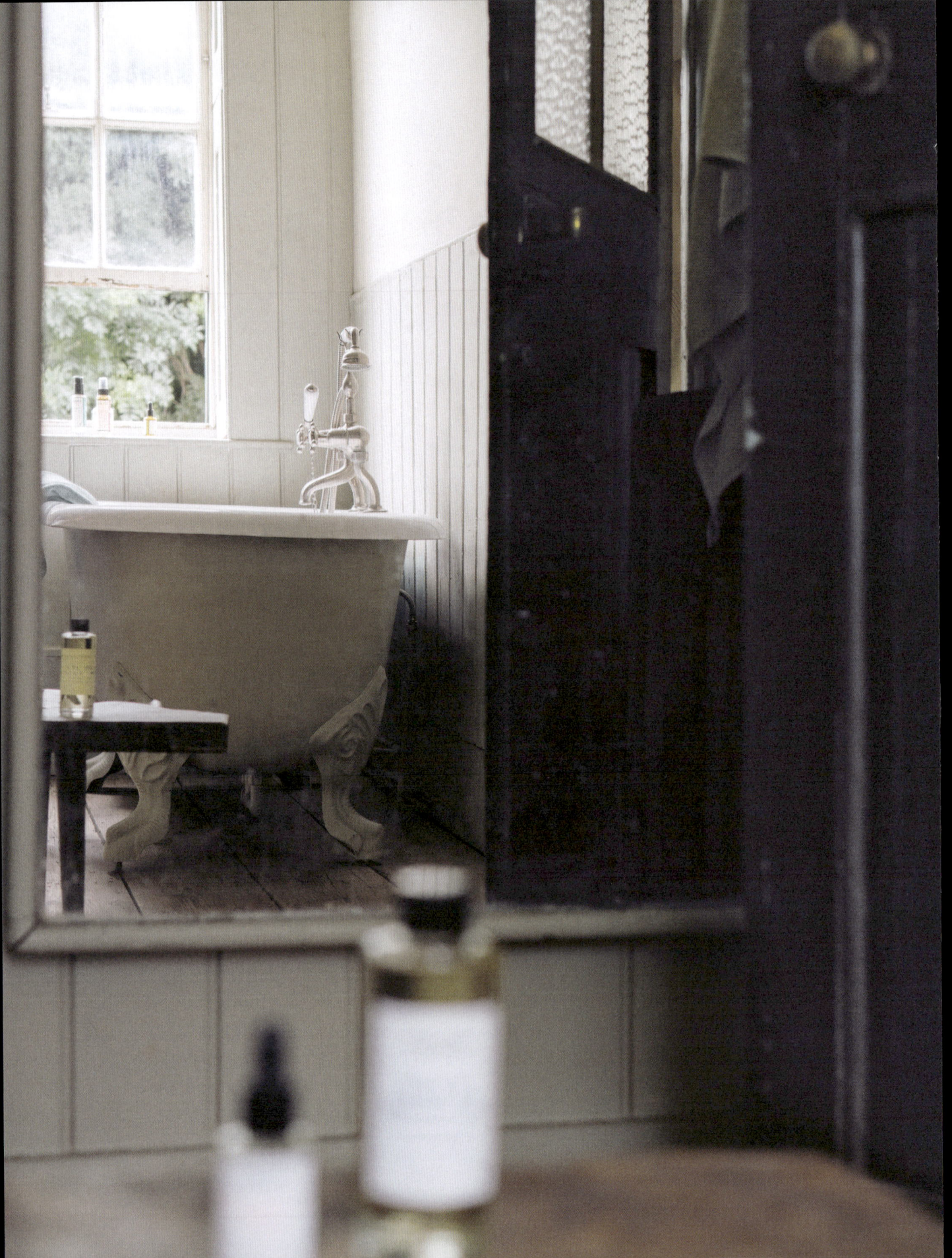

BATHROOM PRACTICE

On average, we spend between 20 and 32 minutes in our bathrooms every day, excluding beauty and make-up time. Bathroom time, which used to be extremely private in most societies – and remains this way for physiological needs – is becoming longer and more visible, propelled by social media content highlighting beauty, skincare and make-up routines.

Bathrooms are becoming increasingly glamorous, welcoming and Instagrammable. You may be among those who use the bathroom in a practical, in-and-out way, or you may find it a peaceful, private and creative place where your self-care flourishes. Either way, you can elevate your bathroom time with simple gestures, turning it into one of your favourite moments in the day.

Leave your phone behind

Unless you're making videos of your practices (in which case, do share them with our team), there is no need to take your phone into the bathroom with you. It's unnecessary in the shower, distracting when you're focusing on your skin and not recommended when you're using the toilet, since prolonging your time sitting on the loo can cause problems such as haemorrhoids.

Time away from your phone will allow you to focus more on yourself. Who needs a screen when there's a mirror showing the most important face in the world?

Shower benefits

There is nothing more intimate than a shower. The water running down your body, either cooling or warming it, the relaxation, the cleanliness, the unique thoughts that come to mind. The majority – 67 per cent – of us have mentally productive shower time. The pensiveness of the moment, channelled properly, can lead to exciting and unique ideas we would be less likely to have in busier, less private contexts.

Another significant percentage of people – most noticeably women – tend to worry in the shower, using the moment on their own to hyperventilate about family, work and other issues that can – and should – wait.

Take this time to perform a breathing exercise, ideal while you let your conditioner work. Massage your scalp with purpose while you apply shampoo, stimulating circulation and relaxing your muscles. Close your eyes and enjoy the soothing sound of water falling.

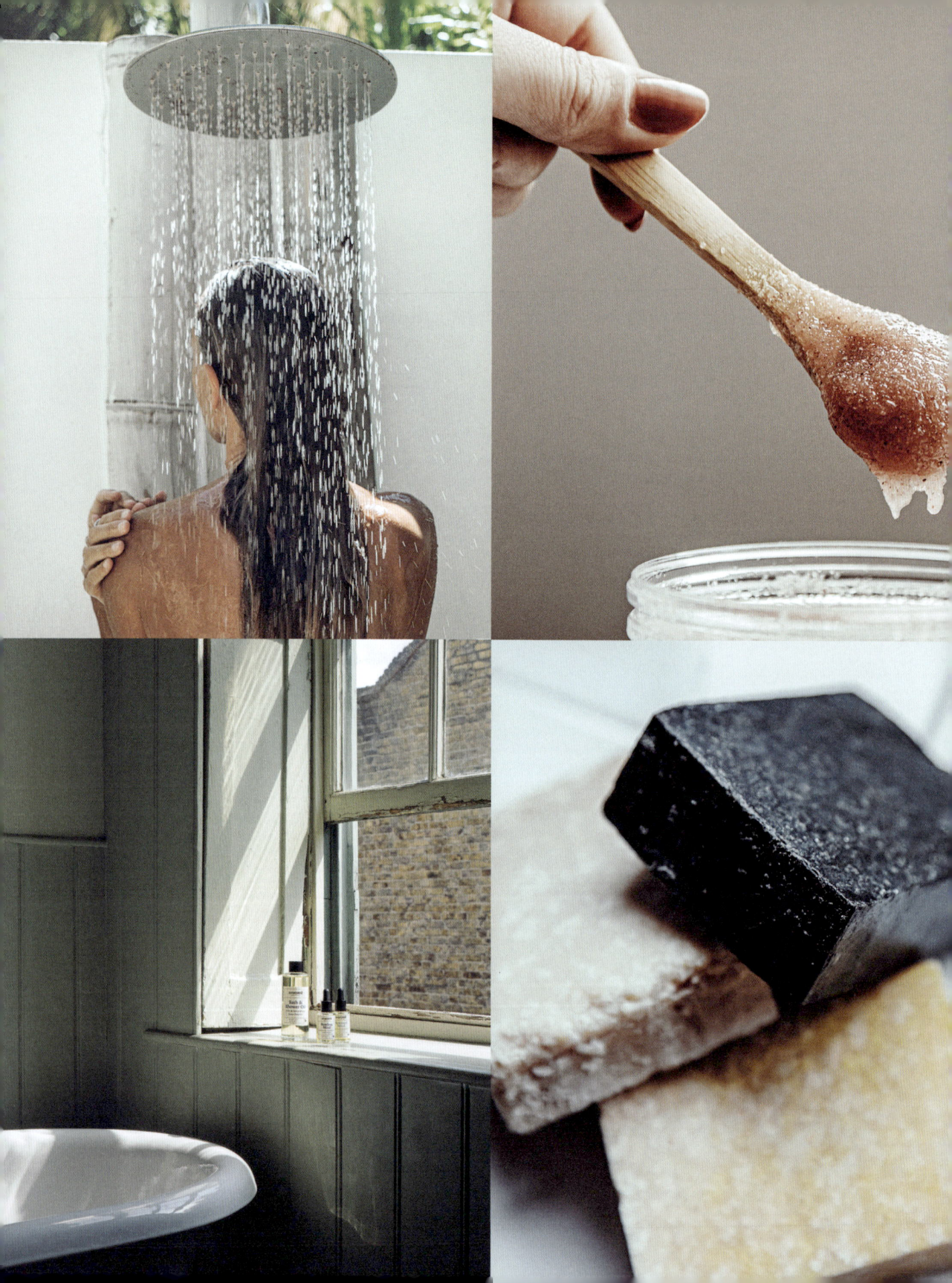

Adjust the water temperature, making sure it's neither too hot nor too cold. The ideal temperature is the one that makes you feel the most comfortable.

Beyond the mirror

Mirrors have always existed. In the past, still water was used as a reflection device. But the mirror as we know it was created relatively recently, in Germany, curiously by an apothecary. Chemist Justus von Liebig applied a thin layer of silver to clear glass and created the first mirror as we would recognize it.

Our bathroom mirrors see the best and the worst of us: when we wake up puffy, with dark circles, when we're coiffed and made-up for a night out, when we admire ourselves, fret about wrinkles and make silly facial expressions.

In our wellbeing practices, we like to think of the mirror as a window to self-love. If you're using it for a skincare routine, make sure you discover every detail of your face. Accept the 'flaws' or make a plan to change them. But don't obsess. It's your face, with all its unique traits, signs of time and features.

Smile at yourself to acknowledge what others see when you're happy. You can even take this time to review some of your expressions away from the judgement of others. Make sure your self-judgement doesn't get in the way.

While you're at it, apply your formulations slowly, with soothing, delicate movements that caress your skin. Massage your facial muscles and exercise them to keep them toned. Love what you see.

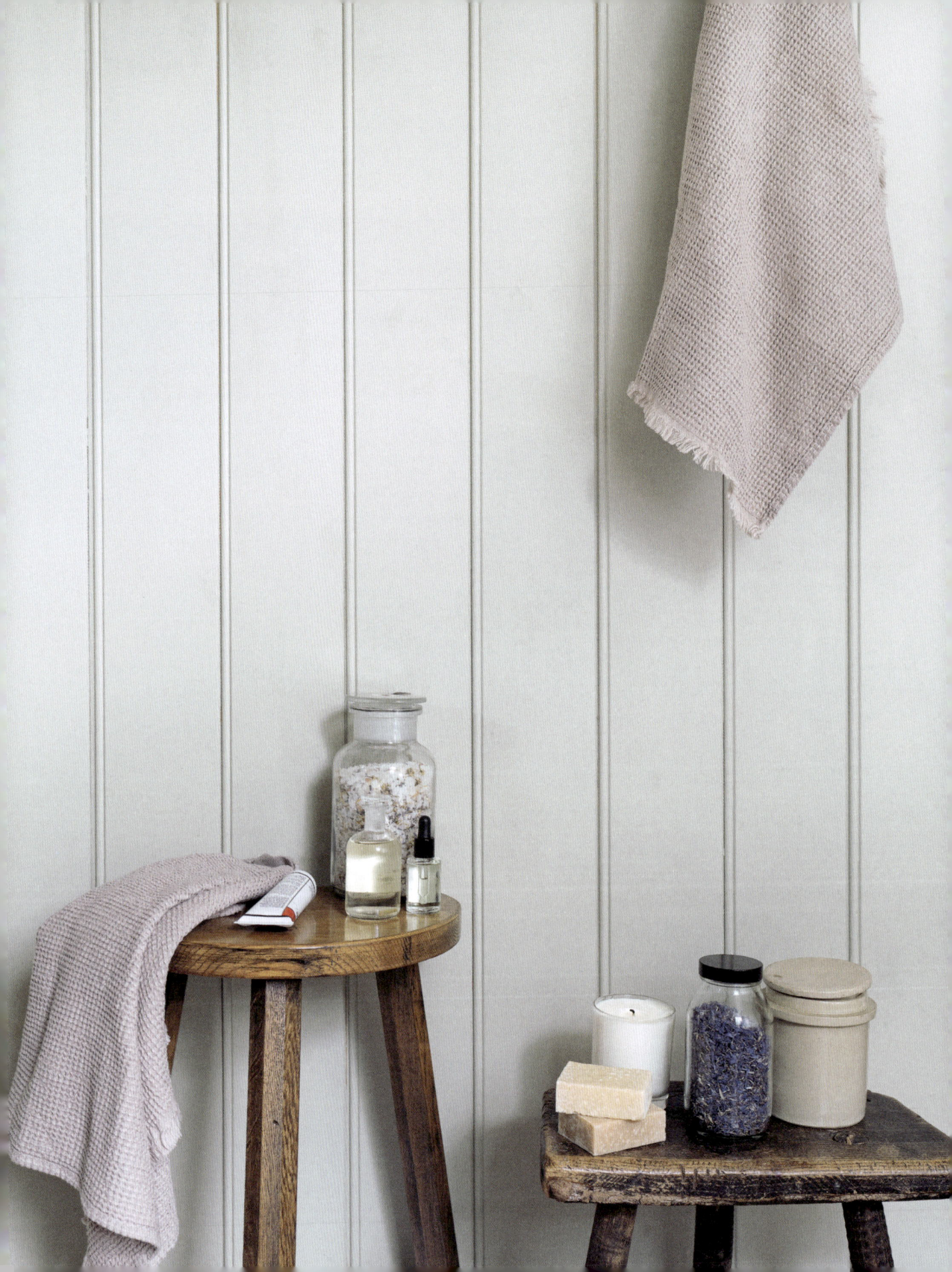

CREATE YOUR HAVEN

Whenever we hold a practice workshop at anatomē, we tend to engage in chaotic conversations around a theme. Everyone has an experience, a habit and plenty of opinions to share. Gradually, we begin to find points in common. That's when we kickstart research to structure a new practice.

When it came to 'Creating Your Haven', the team was sceptical. Why are we discussing interior design or looking at Marie Kondo videos when our work focuses on building the individual?

The answer came in parts. Brendan was discussing the pleasures of a curated home with elements that reflect our personality, alongside post-pandemic ideas of home comfort and wellbeing. Then research showed us our environment – at least the parts we can influence and cultivate – is a fundamental wellbeing pillar. And we can indeed make our living or working spaces support our health and wellness.

The *Cambridge Dictionary* describes the term 'haven' as 'a safe or peaceful place'. We all need one, and most of us already have this place somewhere in our lives. The practice of creating a haven, however, is about taking the safety and peace of your favourite spot and making it conducive to self-care.

In 2020, Americans spent 62 per cent of their waking time at home. In comparison with 2019, when there weren't lockdown measures, the difference is 12 per cent. While we're out and about again, we've learned to spend more time in our homes, investing more than ever in making them better, reflecting our personalities and escaping the outside world.

We all have a favourite area in our homes. It can be the place where the family gathers, where we keep our favourite belongings or where we can be ourselves without interruptions or judgement. In other words, a 'safe and peaceful space'.

To convert your favourite room into a haven or to create one from scratch, we recommend you think about the following points:

- What is my favourite activity when I'm on my own?
- Where does most of my self-care take place?
- How do I imagine a peaceful, safe and comfortable environment?

If you're interested in design, interiors and curating spaces, here's an opportunity to express yourself. If you prefer comfort and the absence of visual information or precious details, here's a chance to declutter and reorganize. If you are indifferent to spaces and believe in detachment from them, focus on the ideal state of mind you want to bring into a room.

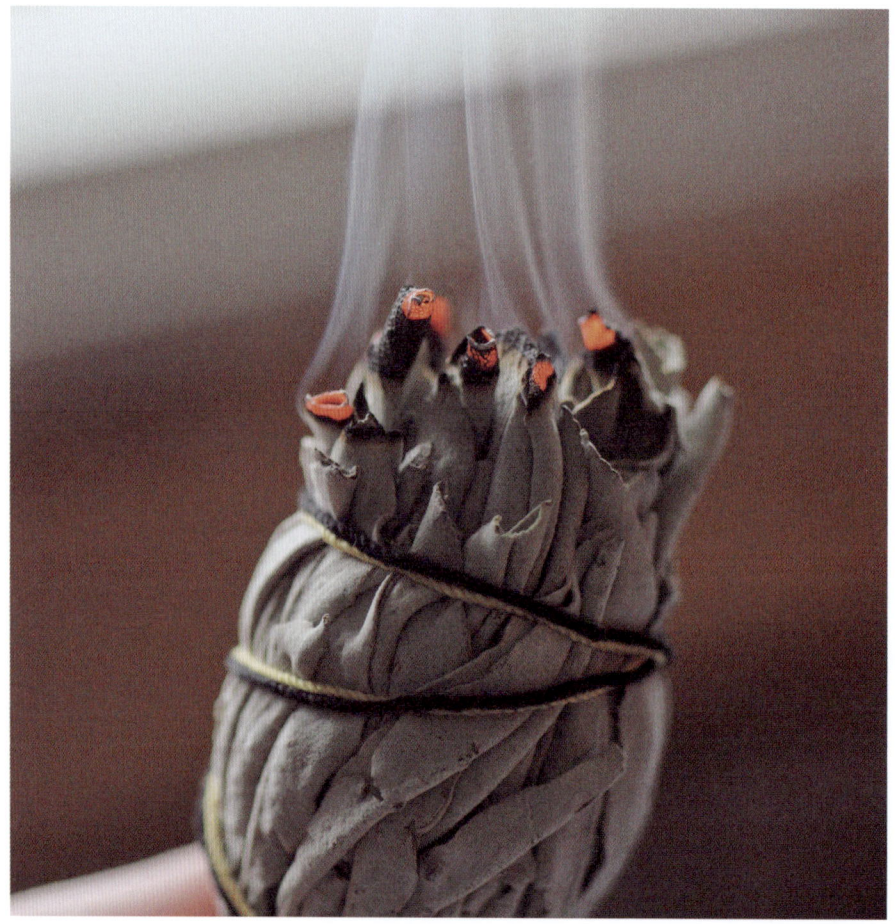

anatomē's
GUIDE TO CREATING YOUR HAVEN

Once you've decided on your dedicated space, it's time to turn it into a wellbeing haven. The following steps will help you create it:

Keep your haven only for pleasurable moments
If you've chosen your bedroom, for example, avoid arguments, work meetings, email-checking or anything that may disrupt your peace. Use it only to sleep, meditate, enjoy intimacy, daydream and for your wellbeing practices. If your haven is a corner in your living room, it works in the same way: good moments only.

Tell others how important that space is to you
Once someone you live with or anyone with access to your space is aware of the importance of that space, they will let you have it, not interfere and know better than to interrupt you when you're enjoying your time there.

Make it spotless
Clean, organize, decorate and make it flawless. Every item should have its place, and this only needs to make sense to you. Paint the walls in a colour that soothes you, choose fabrics for curtains and furniture and make sure to fill it with objects and art that reflect who you are. It's not an interior design challenge nor a room to impress anyone. It's your space to enjoy.

Adjust it to your senses
Start with the temperature. Make sure this place is tempered to your preferences, never too hot or cold. Add a scent that brings you joy – a candle or a diffuser with an essential oil blend aimed at helping you relax, energize, focus or sleep. Add sounds if that works for you, and soundproof it if that's an option.

Manage outside influences
If your haven is a workspace, keep the most creative or rewarding part of your work visible, and stow away anything potentially stressful. During your practice, turn all screens off. If you're in your bedroom, make your bed. If it's the bathroom, check that it's ready to welcome you with only things that promote self-care.

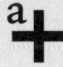

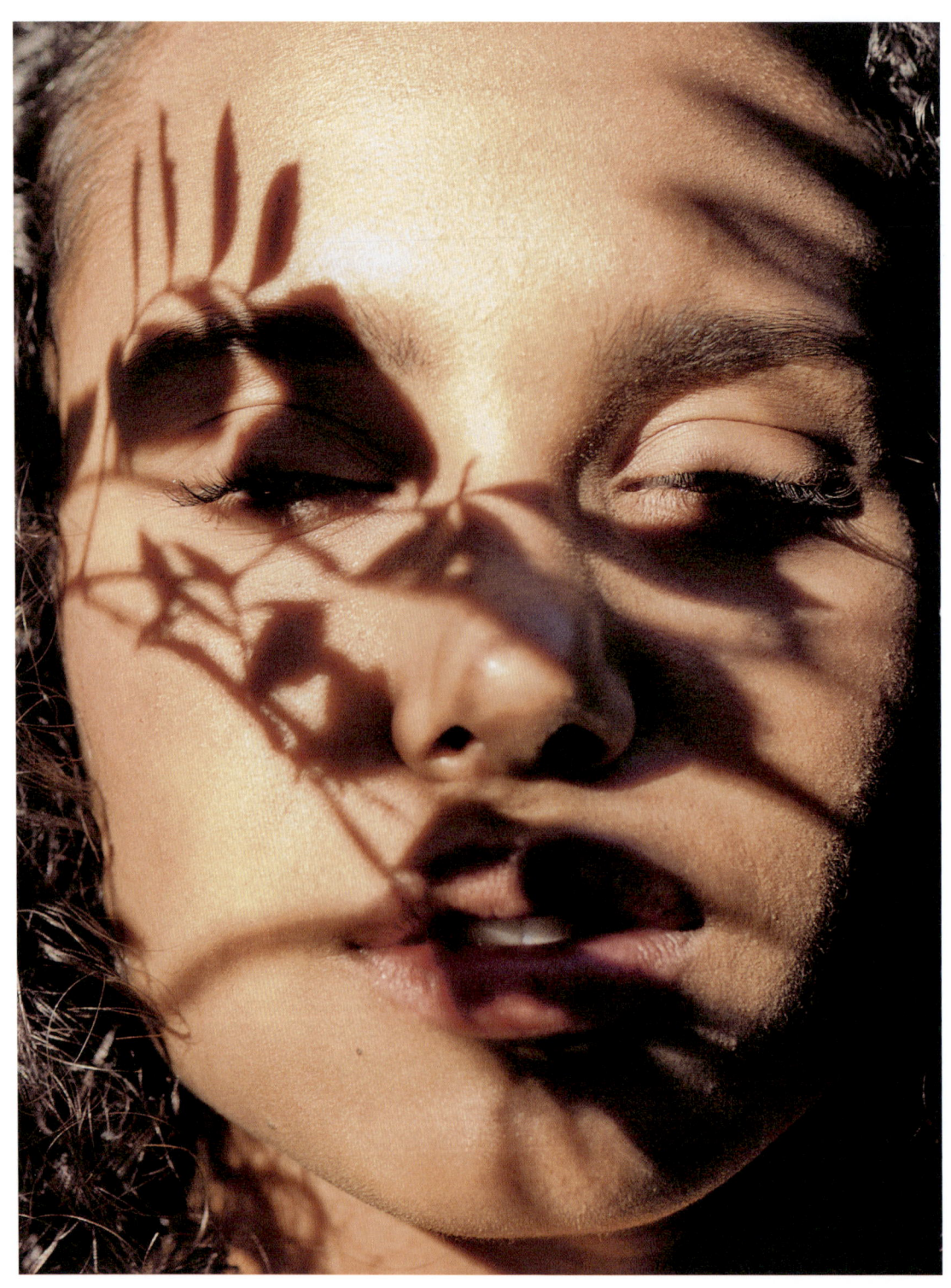

MEDITATE

If you've assessed your wellbeing from a mental health perspective in the past couple of decades – raising questions about stress, lifestyle or insomnia – someone will likely have advised you to try meditation.

We've all met that person: annoyingly bragging about how they meditate every day for at least 5 minutes. They will tell you how wonderful they feel after learning the techniques and how their mindset has changed. They insist you should try it. Again, if you said you have already. And you agree with them to speed up the conversation and change the subject.

Without channelling your meditating friend, we would like to recommend it again. We've incorporated a softcore version of meditation into our wellbeing practices. It's the most efficient way to prepare for a wellbeing practice, helping your brain to slow down, embracing the time you've carved for yourself and allowing your body to benefit from the ingredients. Trust us: it works.

Meditation reached the mainstream around the turn of the millennium, alongside other wellbeing practices such as yoga. The publication of The Power of Now by Eckhart Tolle in 1997, which introduced mainstream readers to mindfulness and meditation practices, helped take meditation to the masses.

Around the same time, the United States saw the rise of yoga studios and classes, which became increasingly popular in the late 1990s and early 2000s as celebrities like Madonna and Sting publicly embraced the practice.

WHAT IS MEDITATION?

Meditation is like the gym, but for the brain: easy to skip, hard to get into and it takes time to show results. The only difference is that while we can immediately spot gym bunnies with toned or muscular physiques, the 'athletes' of meditation aren't visually obvious, potentially making it an even more difficult practice to believe in and embrace.

As such, meditation is mental training. It generates focus, relaxation, presence and awareness. It also involves breathing, posture and commitment. There are three main ways of meditating:

Concentration (focused attention meditation)
It involves focusing your attention (staring, really) on a single, preferably non-moving subject (an object, for example).

Observation (open monitoring meditation)
It's about focusing your attention on the exact moment of the practice: what you're feeling, not letting yourself divert your thoughts to anything else (judgement, for instance).

Awareness
This involves being present in the moment without any interferences – internal or external – focusing, for example, on a specific bodily sensation without judging, explaining or diverting from it.

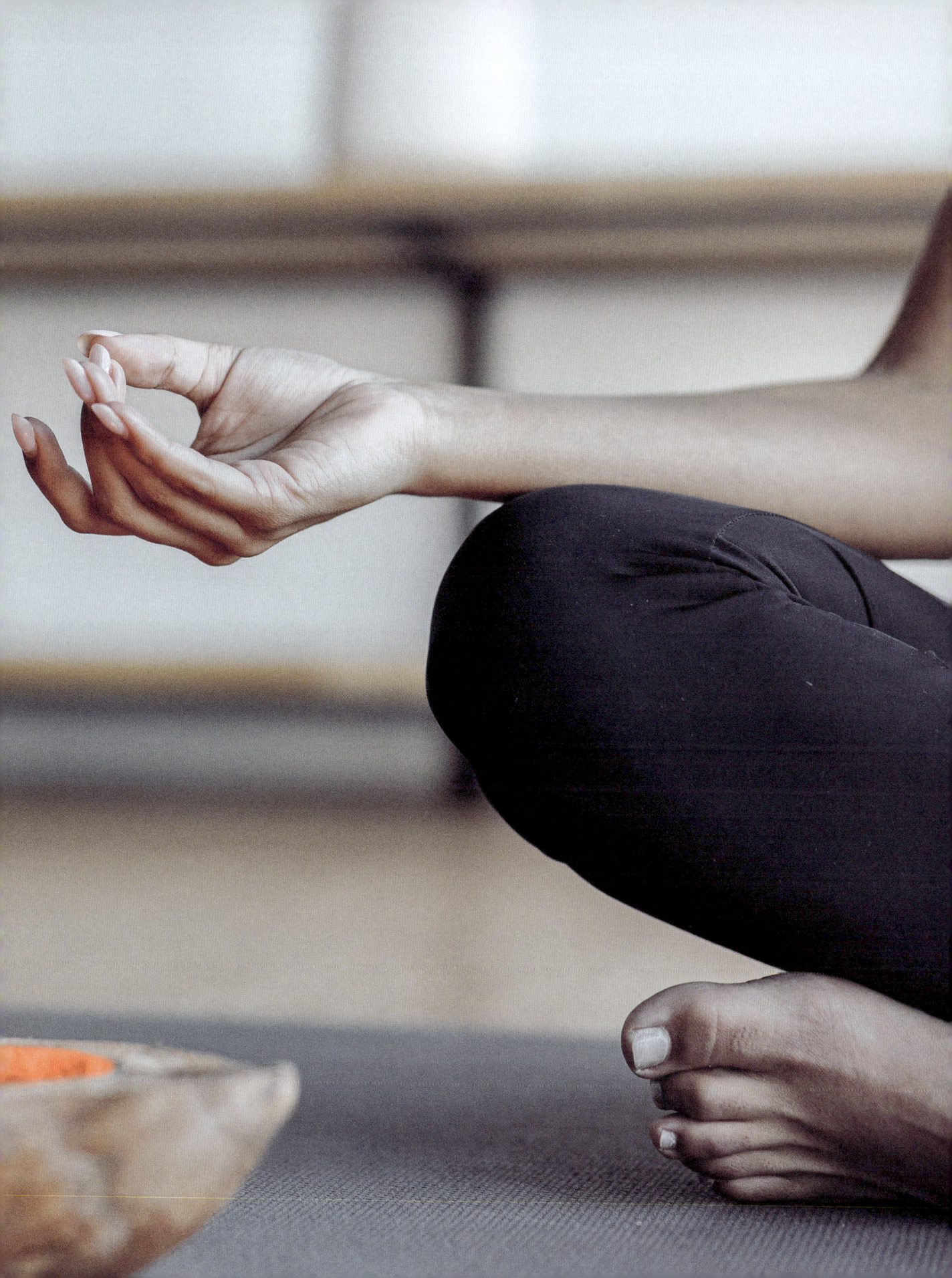

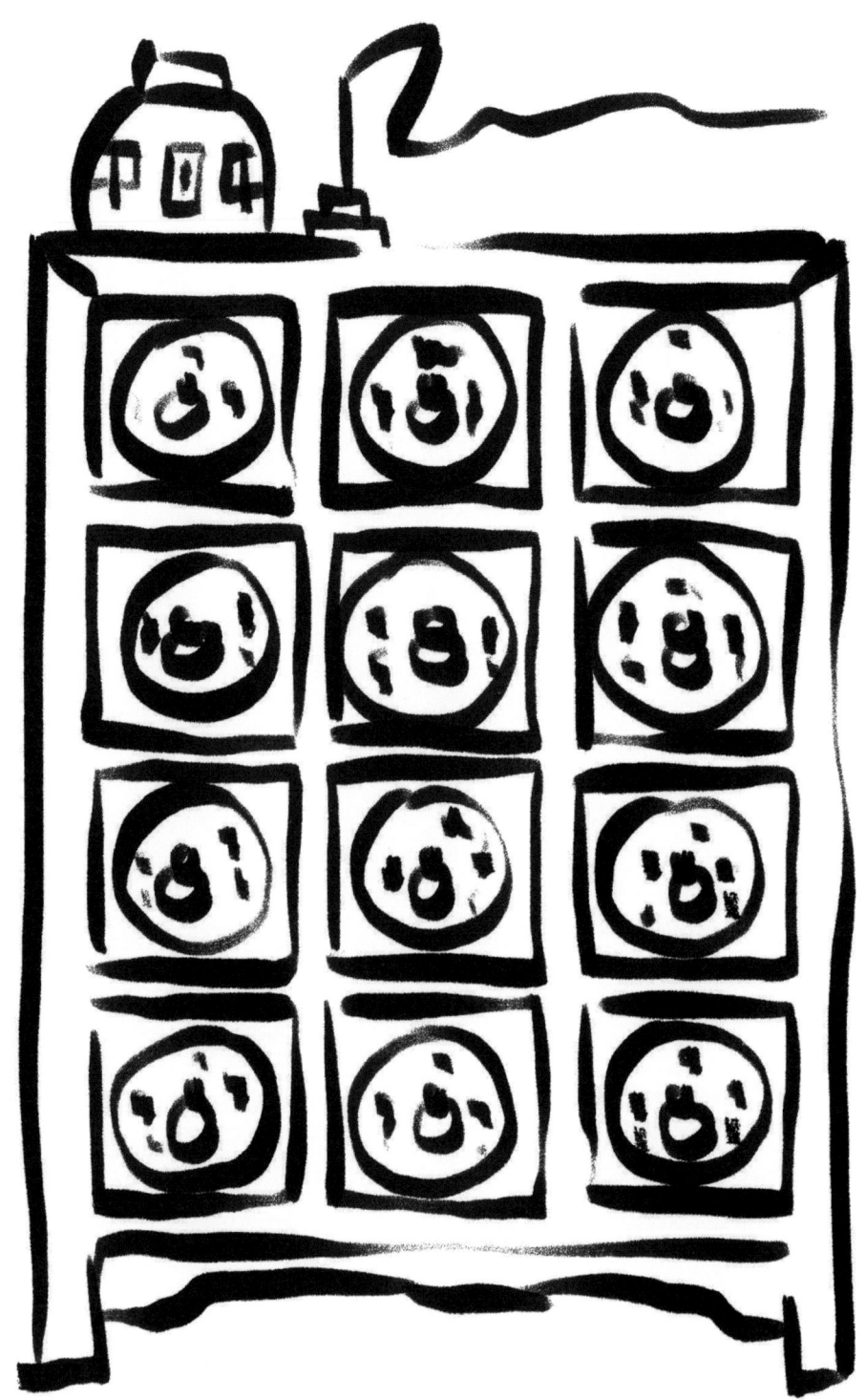

anatomē's
QUICK MEDITATION GUIDE

OK, let's do this. We've created a simplified meditation guide to make it easier for first-timers and support those seeking a light version of meditation.

Find a quiet, comfortable place
There's a common belief that meditation should take place in a minimalist room without any noise, completely sheltered from the world, graced by natural, self-dimming light. Good luck finding that place, and then making it accessible daily. While you want some peace, you should be able to meditate in any reasonably quiet location – outdoors or indoors – where you're less likely to be interrupted.

Find a comfortable position
When it comes to finding the correct position to meditate, there isn't a right or wrong. It's all about being as comfortable as you can. Find a position – sitting or lying – where all your muscles are relaxed. Mind your posture, the tension points you'd like to alleviate, posture vices you need to correct and get to the most stable position you can find. Remember: you'll need to remain in this position for 10 minutes.

Apply a few drops of essential oil onto the palms of your hands and bring your hands close to your nose
It's time to let the scents support your meditation. Your essential oil was likely selected to support a wellbeing need – or because you enjoy its scent. It will anchor your practice, bring you pleasure and, with time, this scent will be associated with your mindful self.

Breathe
Do so slowly and deeply through your nose, allowing your chest and lower belly to rise as you fill your lungs. Let your abdomen expand fully. Now breathe out slowly through your mouth (or your nose, if that feels more natural).

Repeat the breathing, keeping it consistent in timing and intensity. Enjoy.

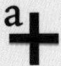

THE ORIGINS OF MEDITATION

Of all subjects approached in this book, meditation is the oldest practice. If we choose to analyze it broadly, considering all types of mental exercise, we could trace meditation back to Neanderthal times, when Neanderthals, according to research, had meditative capacities. To keep our account more concise and limited to meditation with technique, we will go back to 1500 BC.

India
Dhyāna or jhāna, the terms referring to 'mind training', describe a technique close to meditation as we know it today. They were found in records of V*edanta*, an ancient tradition of Hinduism. Buddhist scriptures from a few centuries BC also mention similar practices.

China
References to meditation forms go back to 600 BC. They're linked to writings by Laozi, a Daoist Chinese philosopher. These writings contain terms used for centuries following this time, translated as 'guarding the middle', 'embracing the one', 'guarding tranquillity' and 'embracing simplicity'.

But meditation records exist in many other religions, including Judaism, Islam and Christianity – all of which can be connected to practices we know and are still performed today.

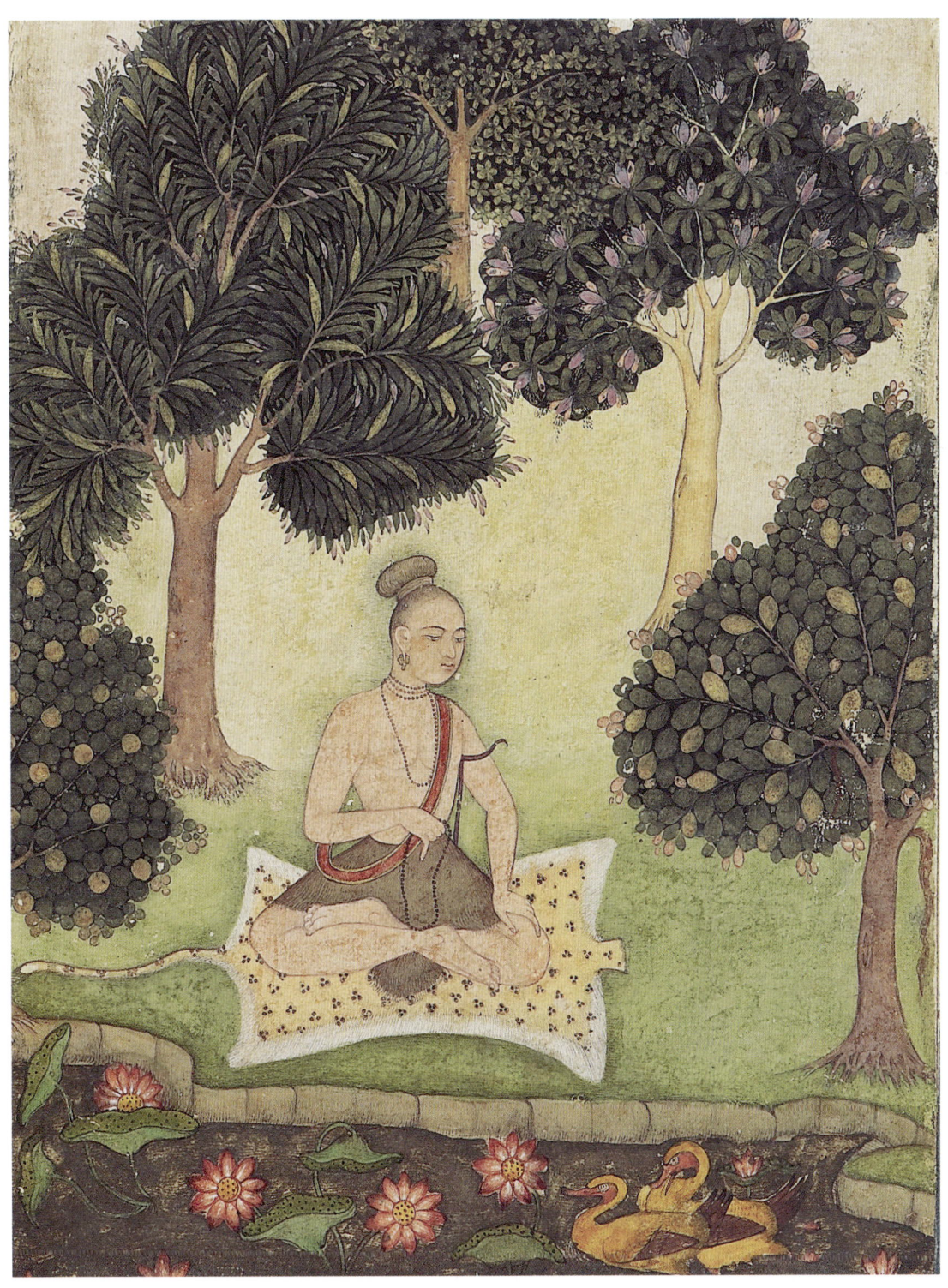

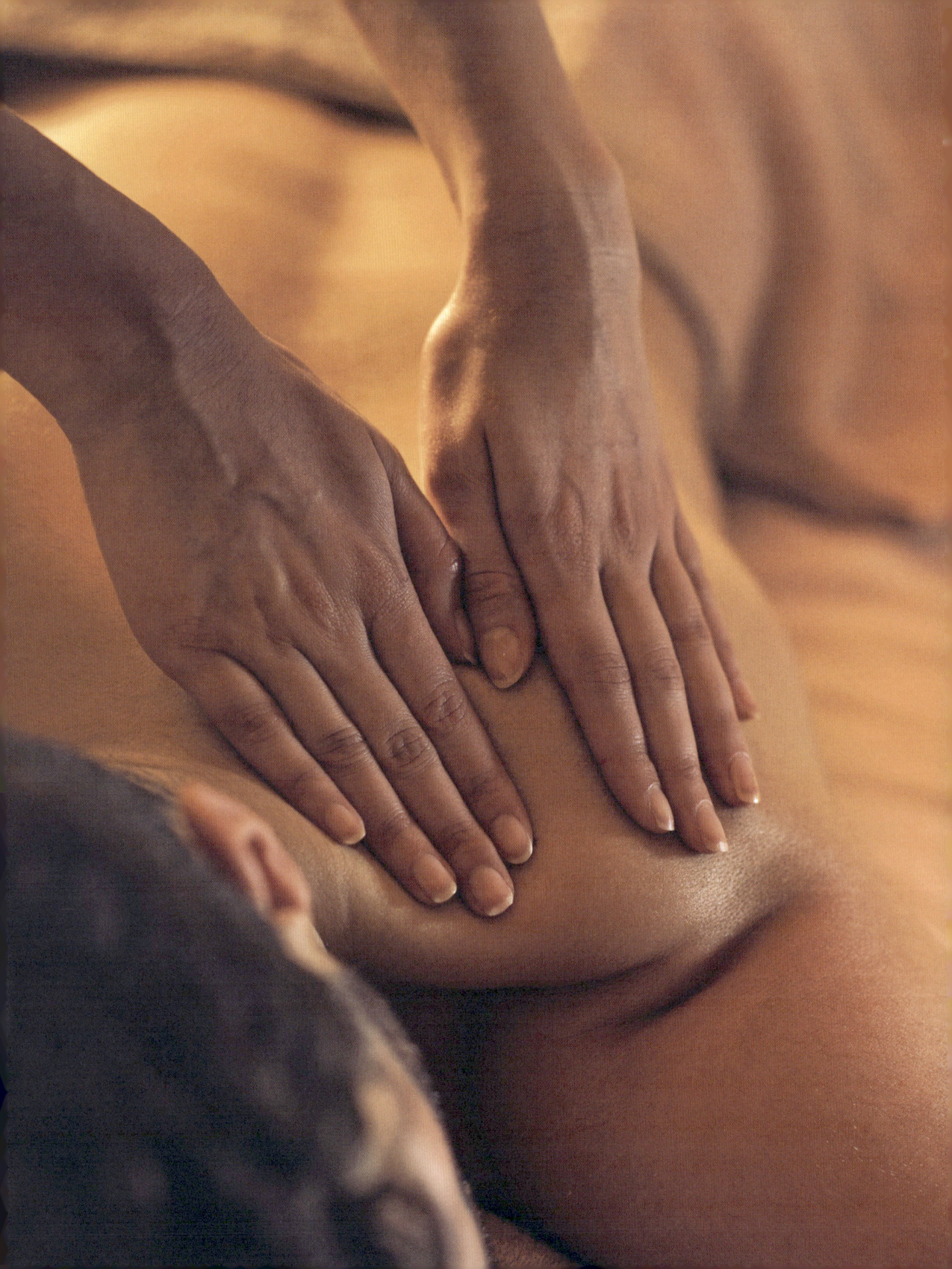

MASSAGE

There's no reason to feel guilty indulging in a massage treatment. In fact, there are many reasons why you need to book a session right now! Studies indicate important physical, mental and emotional benefits from this relaxing therapy.

Most of our daily activities, such as writing, typing on a computer and driving, can cause stress on the body. In particular, our shoulders tend to raise and tighten up when we're busy working. Applying pressure on the soft tissue around your neck, shoulders and back reduces muscular tension and eases day-to-day stress. These parts are constantly holding up our body, so it's no wonder that they feel tense! Here are some key benefits to neck and shoulder massages that aren't just to do with relaxation:

1 Recovery of muscle soreness
Massaging sore areas encourages increased blood flow and oxygen, which helps soothe pain and reduce inflammation. Think of massages as a natural painkiller! After a massage your range of motion will also improve due to the removal of built-up lactic acid, which causes muscle stiffness.

2 Helps reduce migraines
Massages are a natural alternative therapy, without side effects, that help headaches and migraine pain. Massage can relieve muscle spasms and helps blood circulation, which reduces pressure in the head. A study found that patients with ongoing migraines experienced a dramatic reduction in headache pain with neck and shoulder massages.

3 Reduces stress and anxiety
Not only does your body benefit from massages, but your mood elevates too. We carry anxiety in our shoulders, back and neck. Studies found an increase in serotonin and dopamine levels in participants who had massage treatments. When your body is relaxed, so is your nervous system. Your heart rate lowers and so does your breathing, so massages are a useful way to realign your body. Companies like Google offer their employees regular massage treatments because it lessens employee stress and subsequently improves overall job satisfaction. Effects are even stronger when the masseuse uses a massage oil. So use a few drops of your favourite essential oil blend to further invoke calm and relaxation.

4 Strengthens the immune system
If you find yourself not catching a cold after repetitive treatments, you might have to thank your masseuse for that. Participants who took part in a study that consisted of one to two massages a week had an increase of white blood cells and lymphocytes, which are vital for fighting off illnesses and infections.

GET OUTDOORS

When we hear we need to spend more time outdoors, it's usually when we confess to bingeing on a TV series or spending an entire day in bed – at times hungover. It's not easy to switch that off and embrace the wholesomeness of outdoor living. And, for those not naturally interested in spending time outside, the idea of wearing activewear in a park surrounded by fitter people and excessive happiness can be daunting.

Our increasing reliance on technology has prompted us to stay still and indoors more than ever before. We are discovering new forms of enjoyment that don't require the daunting effort of venturing outside and as such, we're building a dangerous habit of rejecting the nourishment of being surrounded by nature, associating it with a lack of dynamism.

The outdoor practice we have created at anatomē takes all that into account. We don't want to turn you into a green t'ai chi practitioner (although it wouldn't hurt), but we can recommend a few steps to make sure you get your weekly dose of greenery, helping your body thrive with all benefits that come from reconnecting with its natural habitat (after all, we were designed to live connected to nature).

Below are all the benefits of outdoor living, with a short and sweet explanation for them, so you can start thinking about it beyond 'just a thought'. Outdoorsiness, even if in small doses, can:

- Help improve your mood, reducing feelings of stress, depression and anger.
- Improve your physical health, particularly if your outside time involves exercise.
- Help you take time out from work and other routines, creating headspace.
- Present social opportunities with a new pool of people, or community, to connect with.

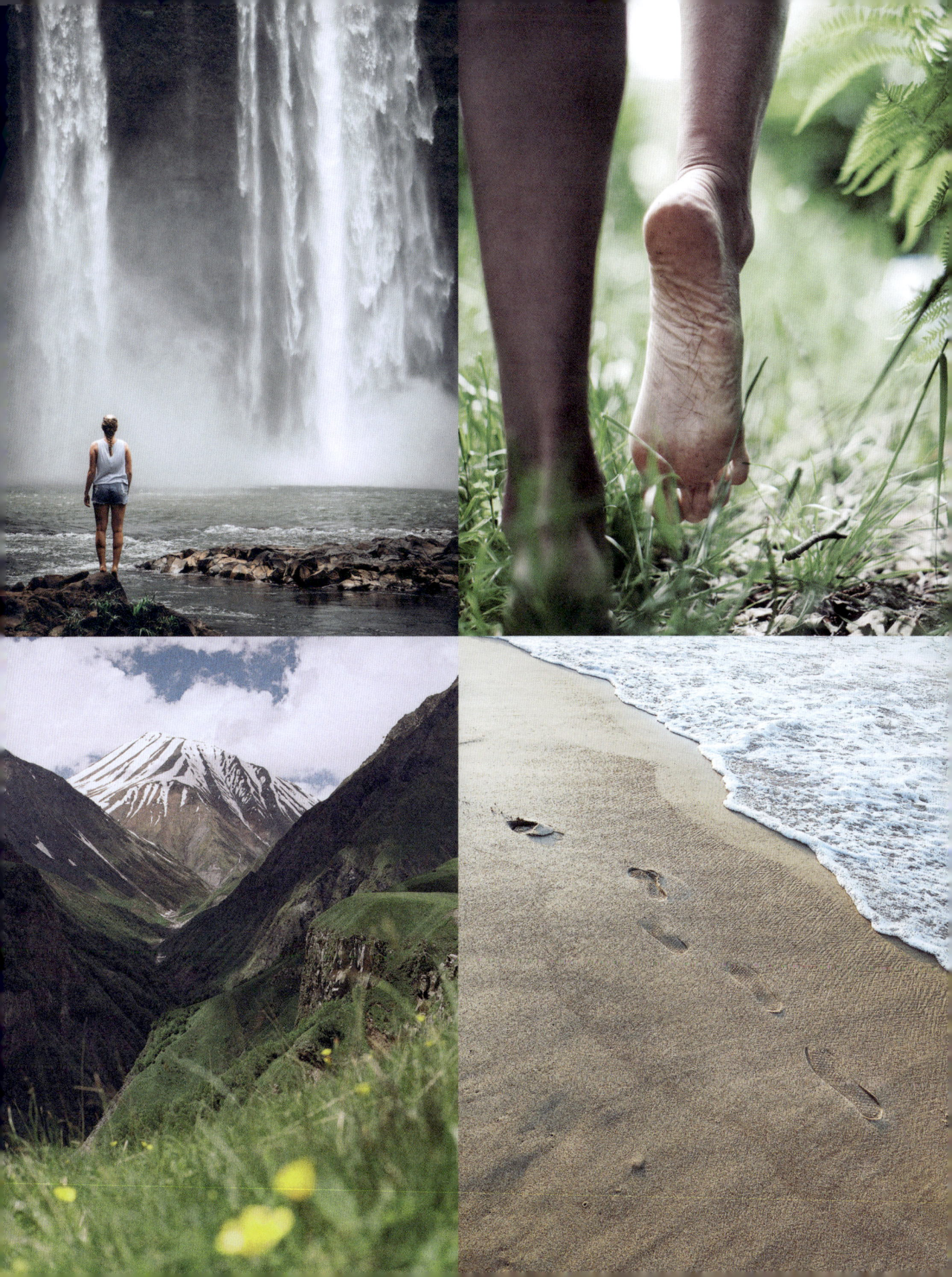

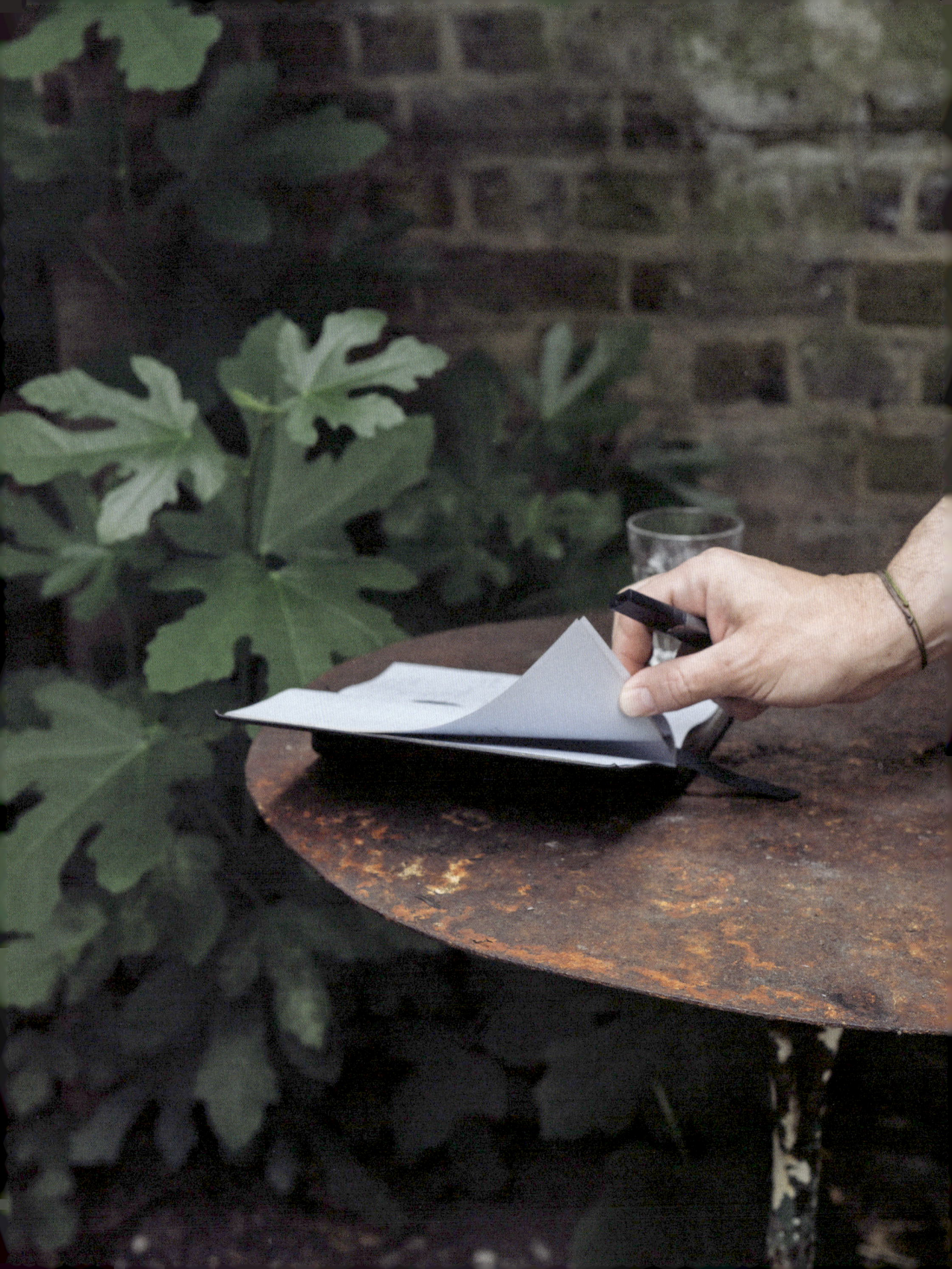

WAYS TO GET OUTSIDE MORE WHILE GETTING ON WITH YOUR ROUTINE

1 Identify commutes you can cycle or walk
Yes, this may take longer than public transport or driving, but if you can make the time to convert some of your journeys into outdoor time, it counts as nature and exercise time. Add a breathing practice, and you're multitasking towards wellbeing.

2 Take outdoor breaks
Whether this means leaving the office for 20 minutes or walking the dog a little longer in the morning, increasing your outdoor time with a healthy break will not only count as nature time but also promote headspace, which is often so scarce in our busy modern lives.

3 If your home has outside space, make it pleasant and desirable to use
Read a book there, enjoy your morning coffee or work outside if you can. If you don't have outdoor space at home, find a green space or a park nearby that you can treat as an extension of your home.

4 Open your windows
This may not be as efficient as going outside, but letting the air circulate – even in colder months – and bringing outdoor freshness into your home is a way of imitating outdoorsiness without committing to outings you're not ready to take. (Make sure you follow this one as last resort or in addition to one of the above.)

FRESH AIR: AN OLD REMEDY

The COVID-19 pandemic made us more aware of the benefits of fresh air, but the idea of ventilation for better health dates from the nineteenth century. At the time, doctors, architects and Florence Nightingale – the nurse who also invented data visualization – began to discuss ventilation and its importance to human health.

Their discussions changed the way buildings were designed – with more windows and ducts to circulate air. The idea was to prevent disease spread. And it did work for airborne infections. Nightingale Pavilions, named after the nurse who influenced the health-focused aspect of hospital building design, consisted of long corridors with windows on both sides, allowing for air circulation and avoiding the spread of diseases.

In the twentieth century, a new therapeutic approach focused on the importance of fresh air and sunshine in the treatment of diseases. Initially applied in hospitals or sanatoriums, it consisted of making patient rooms as sunny and ventilated as possible, helping to treat respiratory infections such as influenza and tuberculosis.

BOTA

HERO
NICALS

THE
POWER
OF
BOTANICALS

Welcome to the world of powerful botanicals that contribute to our wellbeing. These botanicals have been used for centuries to promote physical and emotional wellbeing and play a significant role in modern aromachology practices. The blends, the provenance and the concentration of active compounds within each ingredient make anatomē's formulations unique. Some of these ingredients are known for their benefits in recipes passed from generation to generation, such as herbal teas and infusions. Others have a long history of use by different cultures and civilizations. At anatomē we harness this knowledge – with modern science backing – to create our formulations.

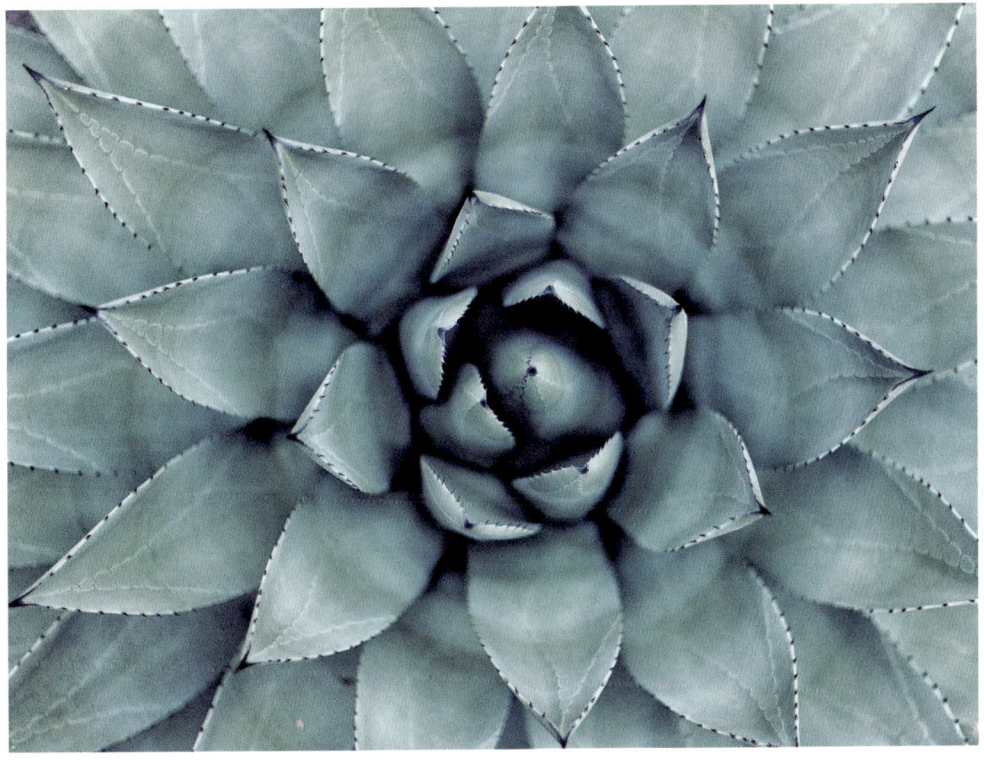

HERO BOTANICALS

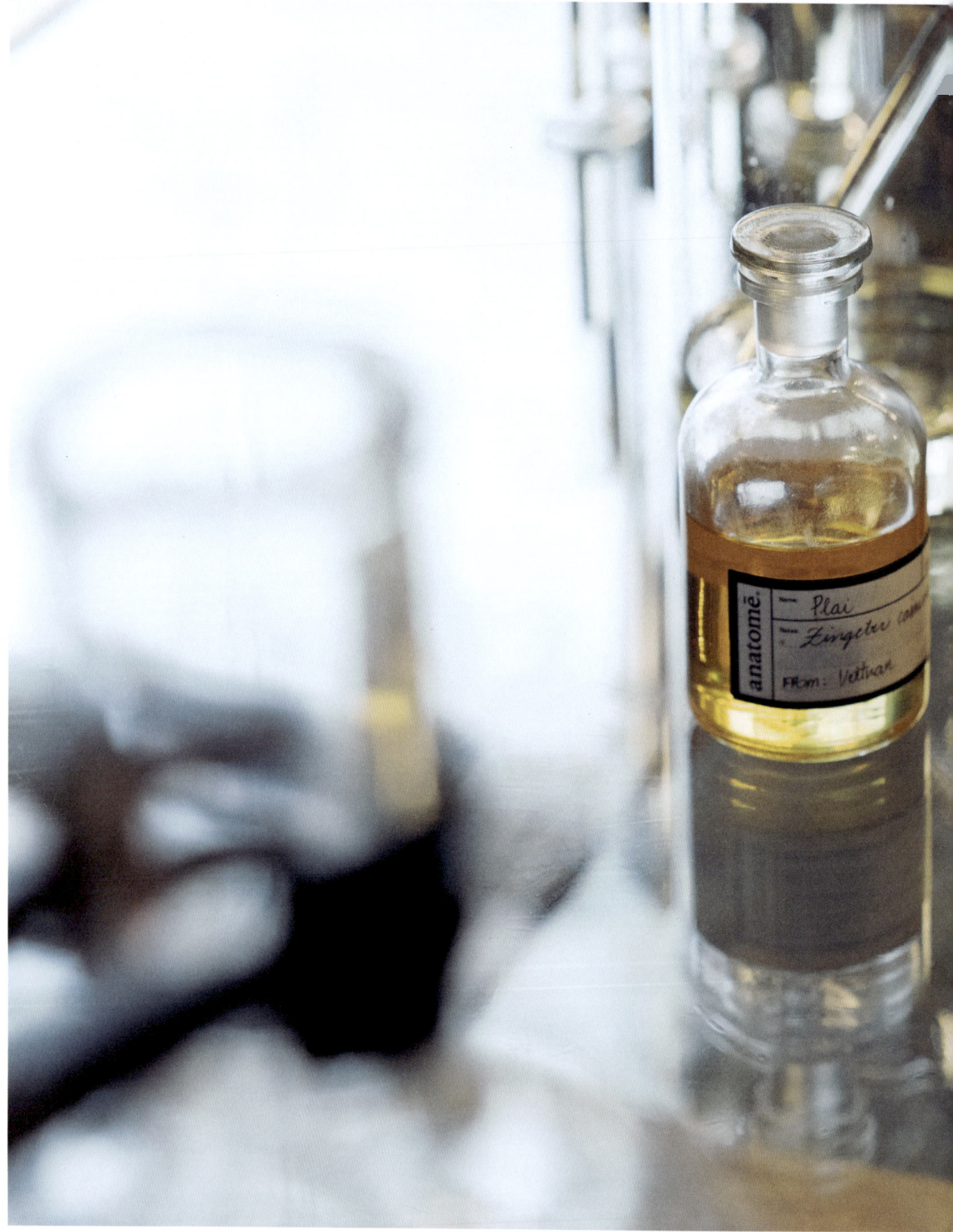

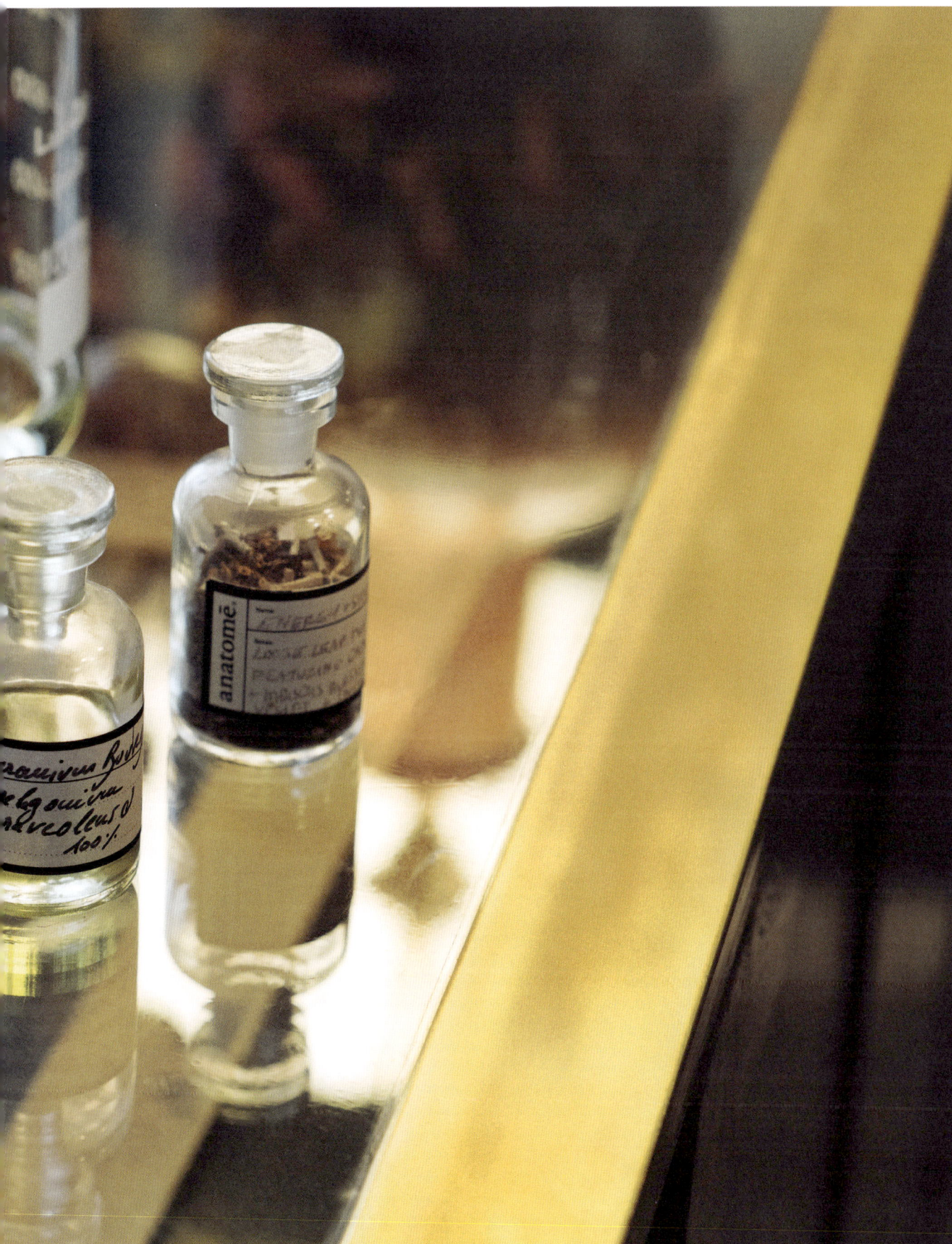

TERPENES – The power of essential oils

Terpenes are produced by plants. This group of organic substances – unsaturated hydrocarbons, to be precise – consist of more than 30,000 different molecules, so when we say anatomē harnesses the power of botanicals, this is what we mean. These extracts or substances are the building blocks of biosynthesis and the main components of many different kinds of plants and flowers' essential oils.

In plants, terpenes and terpenoids aid in the defence against herbivory, disease resistance, attracting mutualists like pollinators and possibly even plant-to-plant communication. Terpenoids also aid in light absorption and photoprotection, plant elongation, membrane permeability and fluidity regulation.

Trivia and background information aside, let's focus on why we harness the power of terpenes for wellbeing. They have been found to have pharmacological effects, and have since been applied in aromachology with success in formulations to sleep, focus and energize.

ADAPTOGENS – Botanicals to support stress

Adaptogens are plants, including mushrooms, that improve general health and assist our bodies in coping with stress, anxiety and exhaustion. We can consume them as tinctures, added to food or drinks, or both. By controlling both physical and emotional stressors, adaptogens help the body regain a stable balance.

To act as an adaptogen, a plant must:
- Not be hazardous when consumed in regulated doses.
- Aid our bodies in overcoming stress.
- Enable our bodies to regain their equilibrium (homeostasis).

What do adaptogens do to the body

The use of adaptogens helps the body achieve balance (homeostasis), speeding up or slowing down the body's chemical processeses.

For instance, an adaptogen will react by lowering high cortisol levels in response to stress. An adaptogen will also raise your body's cortisol levels if you have low cortisol levels and feel persistent weariness. At anatomē we incorporate adaptogens in all of our supplements, alongside scientifically backed ingredients, to support the body as it faces daily challenges. We will come on to them shortly, but these blends are designed to offer solutions to key issues, such as gut health, menopause, hormonal imbalance and fatigue, promising to restore a sense of joy and wellbeing.

anatomē's philosophy is anchored in the choice of botanicals used in each formulation. Comparable to selecting the best ingredients to cook well, formulating with plants, understanding their compounds and selecting the best provenance is a wellbeing gesture.

The next pages summarize our most-valued ingredients, why we use each one, alongside history trivia, to put our ideas into perspective.

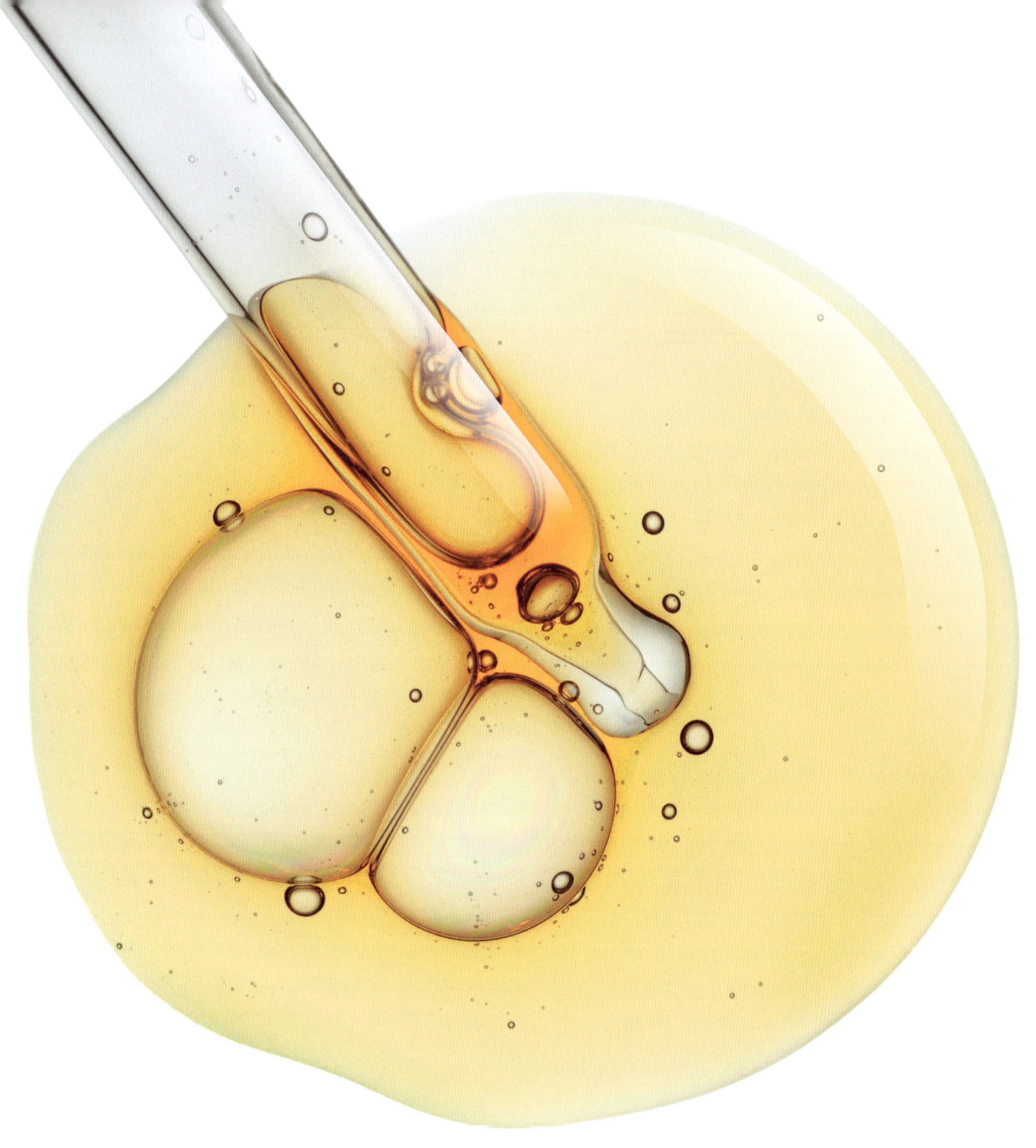

LAVENDER

Lavender oil is one of anatomē's most popular ingredients: it reminds our team and customers of bucolic-scented flower arrangements, taking our minds on vacations in the South of France. Although we love to dream of such lovely images, we apply lavender to our formulations to harness its numerous benefits beyond beauty.

This plant is a member of the mint family, native to the Mediterranean coast, Southern Europe, Africa and South Asia. Aside from its characteristic calming floral scent, lavender oil contains potent chemical components such as linalool, linalyl acetate and camphor that act as anxiety relievers and sedatives, interacting with the brain and nervous system to reduce agitation and restlessness and fight depression. Linalool, linalyl acetate, 1,8-cineole B-ocimene, terpinene-4-ol and camphor help boost GABA, a tranquil neurotransmitter for a restful night's sleep. Reduced GABA activity has been associated with insomnia. One study found that levels were 30 per cent lower in insomniacs than in those who slept a full night.

HISTORY

When Tutankhamun's tomb was opened, in 1922, the explorers found traces of lavender within the remains. And the reports of the time say that one could still detect the powerful scent 3,245 years later.

Romans cooked with lavender, used it as an insect repellent and applied it as an antiseptic when dressing battle wounds.

In England, the ever-so-versatile botanical is one of the nation's oldest perfumes. Queen Elizabeth I enjoyed lavender as a fragrance and as a conserve.

Lavandula angustifolia

Here at anatomē, we celebrate this botanical's pain-relieving and sedative qualities, as well as its sweet, calming scent. Lavender's soothing aroma and efficacy in relieving anxiety and pain inspired our relaxing bath salts and massage oil. We also use it in our skincare products, harnessing its ability to help renew skin cells, control pores and rejuvenate the skin. Due to the complexity of this blend of chemicals reacting with the olfactory system, an intentional scent association and rituals that induces relaxation can be built over time. Choose Cornish, Provençal or Himalayan lavender, due to the high concentrations of linalyl acetate and linalool in these varieties.

Wellbeing challenge: RESTLESSNESS
Support ingredient: LAVENDER

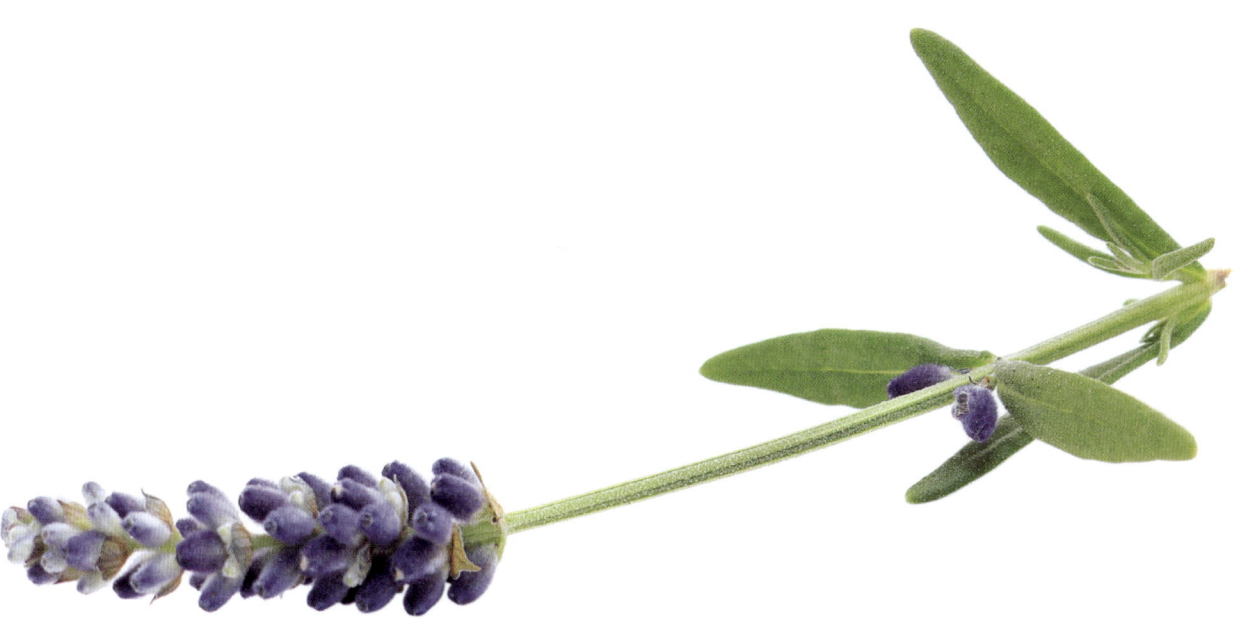

MAY CHANG

May chang is a small tropical tree native to China and Southeast Asia, particularly in Indonesia. May chang oil is extracted from the tree's fruit, and it has a fresh, citrusy aroma with hints of lemongrass and lemon verbena. It's a popular ingredient in aromatherapy due to its uplifting and energizing qualities.

May chang contains high levels of citral, a natural compound found in lemongrass and other citrus fruits. Citral has a variety of benefits, including antibacterial, anti-inflammatory and antifungal properties. May chang oil is also believed to help reduce stress and anxiety, boost mood and promote relaxation.

In addition to its aromatherapy benefits, may chang is also commonly used in skincare products due to its ability to help balance oily skin and reduce the appearance of blemishes. It's often found in toners, serums and moisturizers, as well as in soaps and other personal care products.

HISTORY

May chang has a long history of use in traditional Chinese medicine. Its leaves and fruits were used to treat a variety of conditions, including asthma, indigestion and muscle aches. The plant was also used to relieve stress, anxiety and fatigue, with its fresh and uplifting scent being highly valued. In more recent times, may chang has gained popularity in aromatherapy and natural skincare, where it is known for its cleansing and rejuvenating properties.

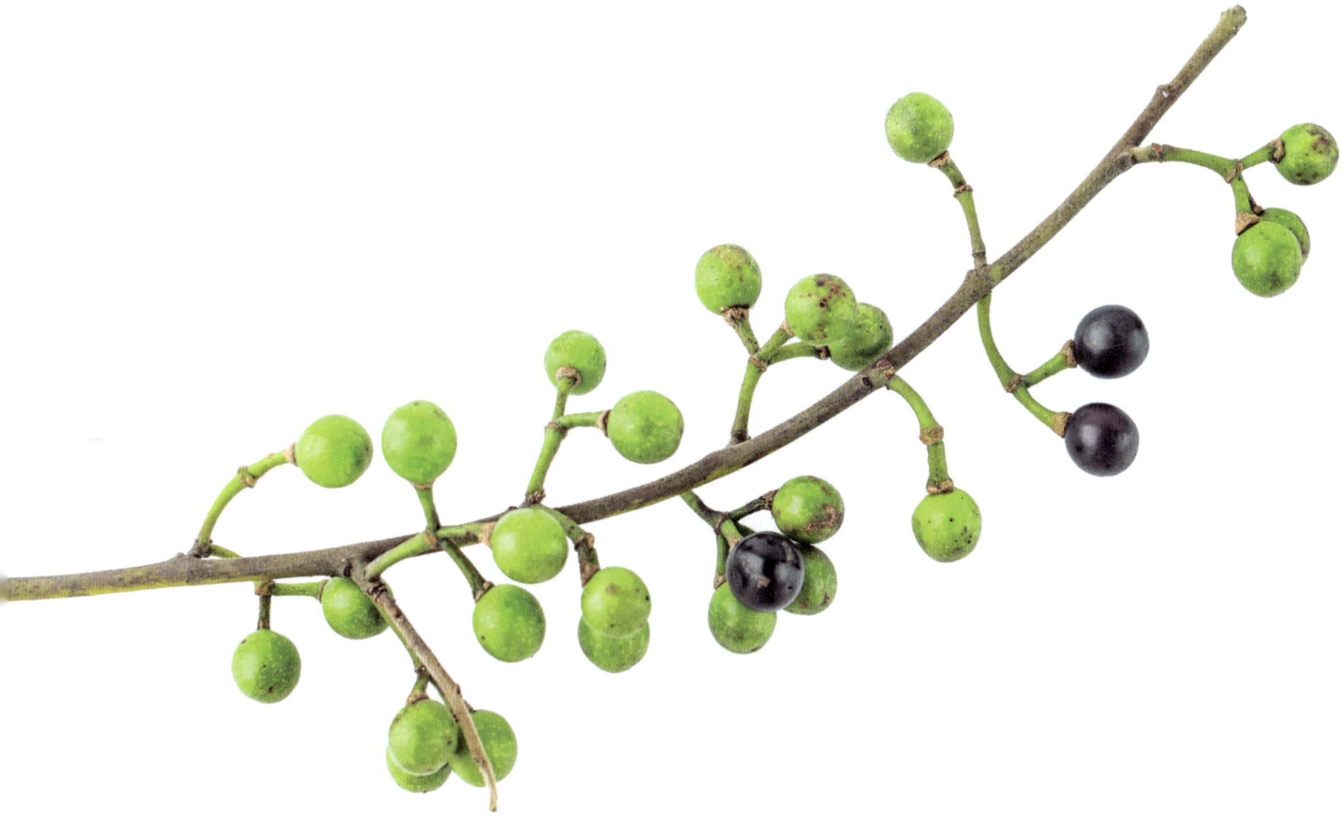

Litsea cubeba

May chang oil has many benefits, from improving skin health to relieving stress and boosting energy levels. It contains a high citral concentration, making it an effective natural treatment for acne and other skin conditions. This oil can also help reduce stress and anxiety, promoting a sense of calm and relaxation. Its uplifting scent has a stimulating effect on the mind, increasing mental clarity and focus. It is also believed to positively impact the respiratory system, helping to alleviate symptoms of colds, flu and other respiratory infections. May chang oil is known to have a refreshing and rejuvenating effect on the body, promoting vitality and wellbeing.

Wellbeing challenge: LOW MOOD
Support ingredient: MAY CHANG

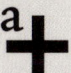

GERANIUM BOURBON

Close your eyes and imagine a lush garden overflowing with colourful blooms. The sweet scent of Geranium bourbon fills the air, transporting you to a place of tranquillity and peace. This beloved flower – an anatomē favourite – has been prized for centuries for its intoxicating fragrance and therapeutic properties.

Geranium bourbon oil has a sweet and floral fragrance with a hint of mint. It is used in aromatherapy for its calming and balancing effects on the mind and body. Geranium oil has been shown to have antibacterial and anti-inflammatory properties, making it a popular ingredient in skincare products. Additionally, it has been found to promote wound healing and reduce pain. Its chemical constituents, such as citronellol and geraniol, are responsible for these therapeutic effects. Geranium oil is often combined with other essential oils to enhance its benefits, and it is generally considered safe for use in aromatherapy and skincare.

HISTORY

Ancient Egyptians used geranium to balance the body's natural energy and help treat ailments. The plant's medicinal properties were later introduced to Europe by Arab traders in the seventeenth century. During the Victorian era, geranium became a popular perfume scent and was even used in traditional medicines. Geranium essential oil is still widely used in aromatherapy and skincare products due to its balancing, calming and uplifting effects on the mind and body.

Pelargonium roseum

Geranium bourbon essential oil is often used in aromatherapy to help improve mood imbalances, such as anxiety and depression. Scientific studies have shown that geranium oil has anxiolytic and antidepressant effects on the brain, which can help to reduce feelings of stress and anxiety. It is believed that the active components in geranium oil work by modulating the levels of neurotransmitters like dopamine and serotonin in the brain, which are associated with mood regulation. Geranium oil has also been shown to have anti-inflammatory and antioxidant properties, which may contribute to its beneficial effects on mood and mental health.

Wellbeing challenge: MOOD INBALANCE
Support ingredient: GERANIUM BOURBON

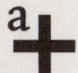

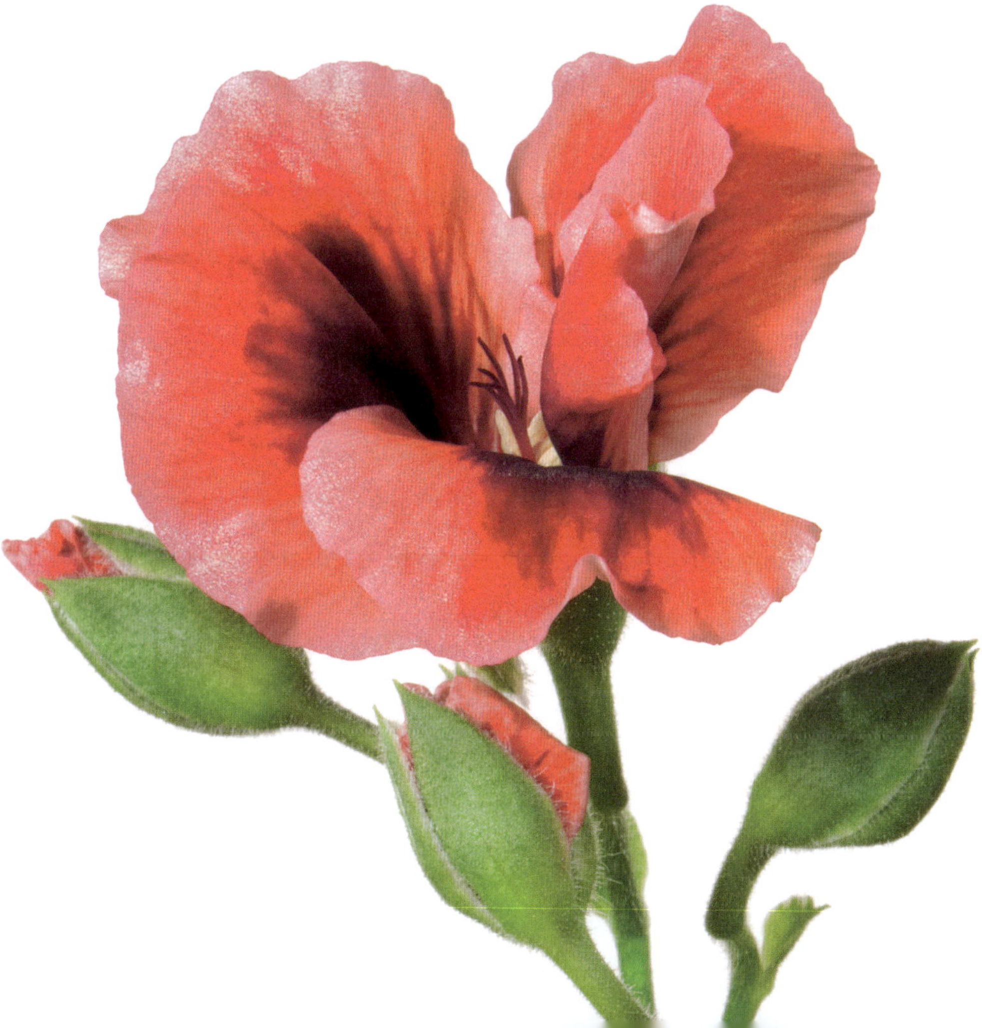

SOMALI FRANKINCENSE

The aroma of Somali frankincense allows us to experience the mystic of ancient rituals. Close your eyes and imagine being transported to the ancient Middle East, surrounded by this precious resin's warm, woody and slightly citrusy scent. The smoky aroma of burning incense fills your nostrils, creating a sense of calm and relaxation. You feel as though you are in a place of deep spiritual significance, where the air is thick with the presence of a higher power.

This ingredient, also known as *Boswellia Frereana*, is a type of resin obtained from trees native to Somalia. It has been used for centuries in traditional medicine and religious ceremonies. Studies have shown that the essential oil extracted from the resin contains a high amount of alpha-pinene. This compound has anti-inflammatory and anti-anxiety properties. Inhaling the oil can help promote relaxation and reduce stress levels, making it a popular choice for aromatherapy. It has also been found to have wound-healing properties, making it useful in topical applications. Its pleasant, woody aroma and therapeutic benefits make it a sought-after ingredient in many natural health and beauty products.

HISTORY

Somali frankincense has a rich and storied history that dates back thousands of years. It was a prized commodity in ancient times, traded along the spice routes that crisscrossed the Middle East and Africa. It was used in religious ceremonies, as a perfume and medicinal preparations. Somali frankincense was so valuable that it was a known gift to royalty. Today, it remains an integral part of traditional cultures thanks to its many health benefits. Its rich history and cultural significance continue to make it a sought-after ingredient in perfumes, cosmetics and aromatherapy products.

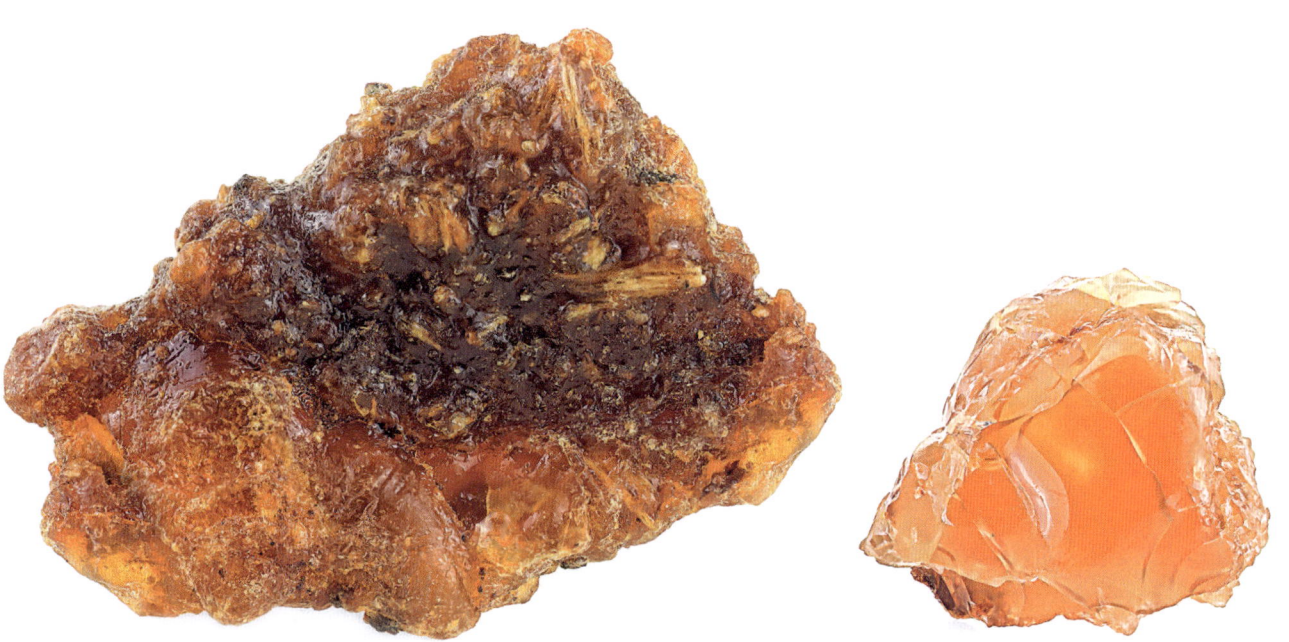

Boswellia Frereana

Somali frankincense has been used for centuries to calm and focus the mind. Modern science has confirmed its benefits for those who struggle with an overactive mind, including symptoms of anxiety and depression. The resin contains boswellic acids with anti-inflammatory properties that help alleviate stress and promote relaxation. Additionally, Somali frankincense has been shown to increase activity in the limbic system, which regulates emotions and mood. This increased activity can lead to a more balanced emotional state.

Wellbeing challenge: OVERACTIVE MIND
Support ingredient: SOMALI FRANKINCENSE

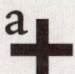

ROMAN CHAMOMILE

Picture yourself in a field of vibrant blue flowers, swaying gently in the breeze. Each petal holds the essence of a calming oasis, transporting you to a world of tranquillity. As you breathe in Roman chamomile's delicate fragrance, you can feel your worries melt away, and a sense of peace wash over you.

Roman chamomile, scientifically known as *Chamaemelum nobile*, is a flowering plant native to Western Europe and North Africa. It has a sweet, fruity scent, and it's known for its calming properties. Its essential oil is widely used in aromatherapy to promote relaxation and improve sleep quality. In addition to its calming effects (the most important of its benefits for anatomē), Roman chamomile is also known for its anti-inflammatory and anti-bacterial properties, making it a popular natural remedy for skin conditions and digestive issues. In cooking, it performs as a flavouring agent, especially in teas and baked goods, and its flowers are also used to produce perfumes and cosmetics.

HISTORY

In ancient Egypt, Roman chamomile was considered a sacred herb with healing properties. The Egyptians used it in cosmetics, medicine, embalming and as an offering to the gods. The Romans later adopted chamomile for its medicinal properties, calling it 'the plant's physician' because it seemed to heal any plant growing nearby. Roman chamomile is still highly regarded for its calming and soothing properties, applied in aromatherapy and skincare.

Chamaemelum nobile

Roman chamomile oil contains an array of bioactive compounds, including chamazulene, α-bisabolol and apigenin, which have antiseptic and anti-inflammatory properties. When diffused or applied topically, Roman chamomile oil is known for its calming and relaxing effects on the body and mind, making it a popular choice for promoting sleep and reducing anxiety. It also soothes skin irritation and promotes wound healing due to its antiseptic properties.

Wellbeing challenge: INTERRUPTED SLEEP
Support ingredient: ROMAN CHAMOMILE

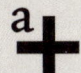

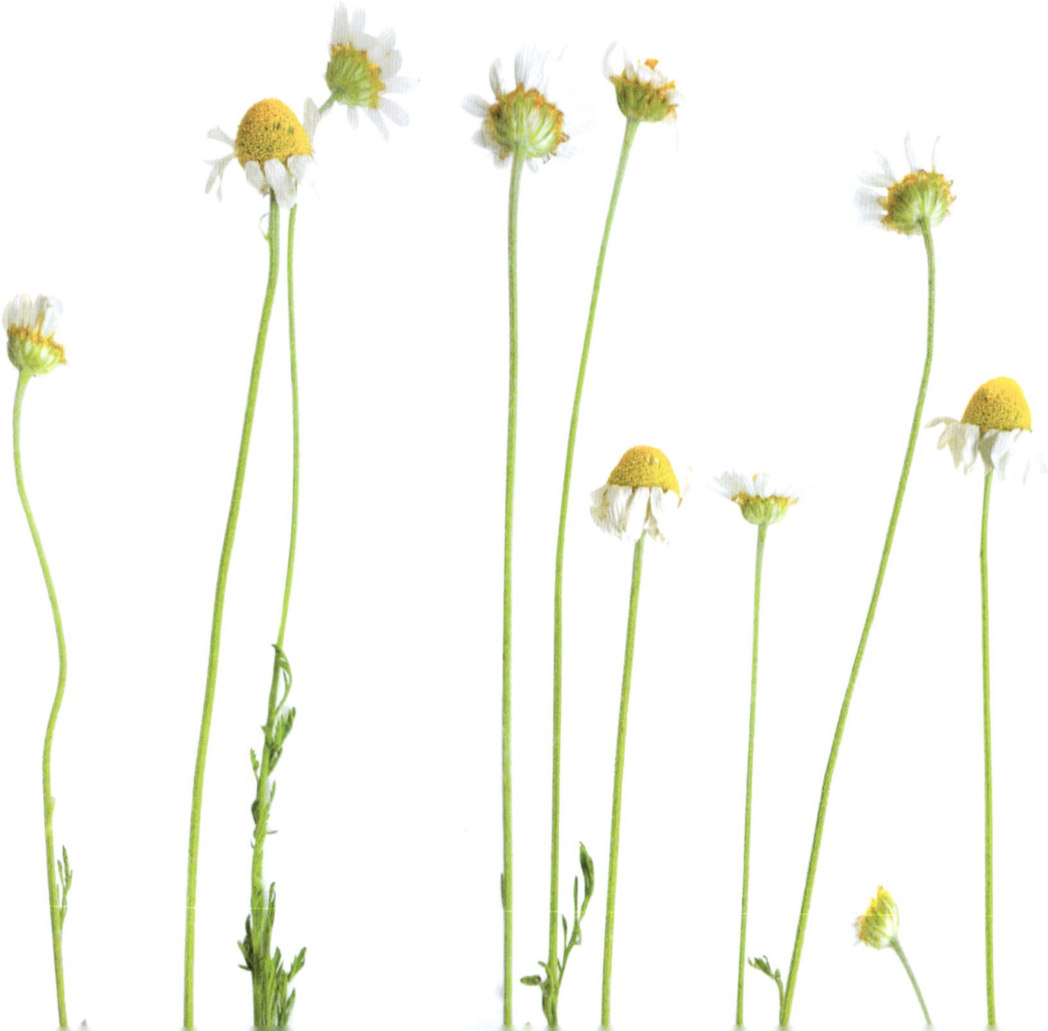

WAKAME

A type of Japanese seaweed, wakame is like an underwater forest, swaying gently in the currents of the Pacific Ocean. Its long, delicate fronds dance in the water, creating a mesmerizing, relaxing and sleep-inducing sight alone. With its earthy, umami flavour and nutrient-rich composition, wakame has been a staple of Japanese cuisine for centuries.

Scientifically known as *Undaria pinnatifida*, wakame is a type of brown seaweed native to the Pacific Ocean. It is rich in nutrients such as iodine, calcium and magnesium, as well as antioxidants and omega-3 fatty acids. Wakame supports thyroid function, improves digestion and reduces inflammation. It is often used in soups, salads and sushi rolls and as a natural flavour enhancer in Japanese cuisine. In addition to its culinary uses, wakame features in skincare products for its moisturizing and anti-ageing properties.

HISTORY

The history of wakame is closely tied to the culture and cuisine of Japan. This seaweed has been used in Japanese cooking for over a thousand years and has played a significant role in developing Japanese cuisine. In ancient times, it was used as a food source for samurai warriors during battles due to its high nutritional value. Today, wakame is a beloved ingredient in many traditional Japanese dishes, such as miso soup and seaweed salad, and has gained popularity worldwide for its unique flavour and health benefits.

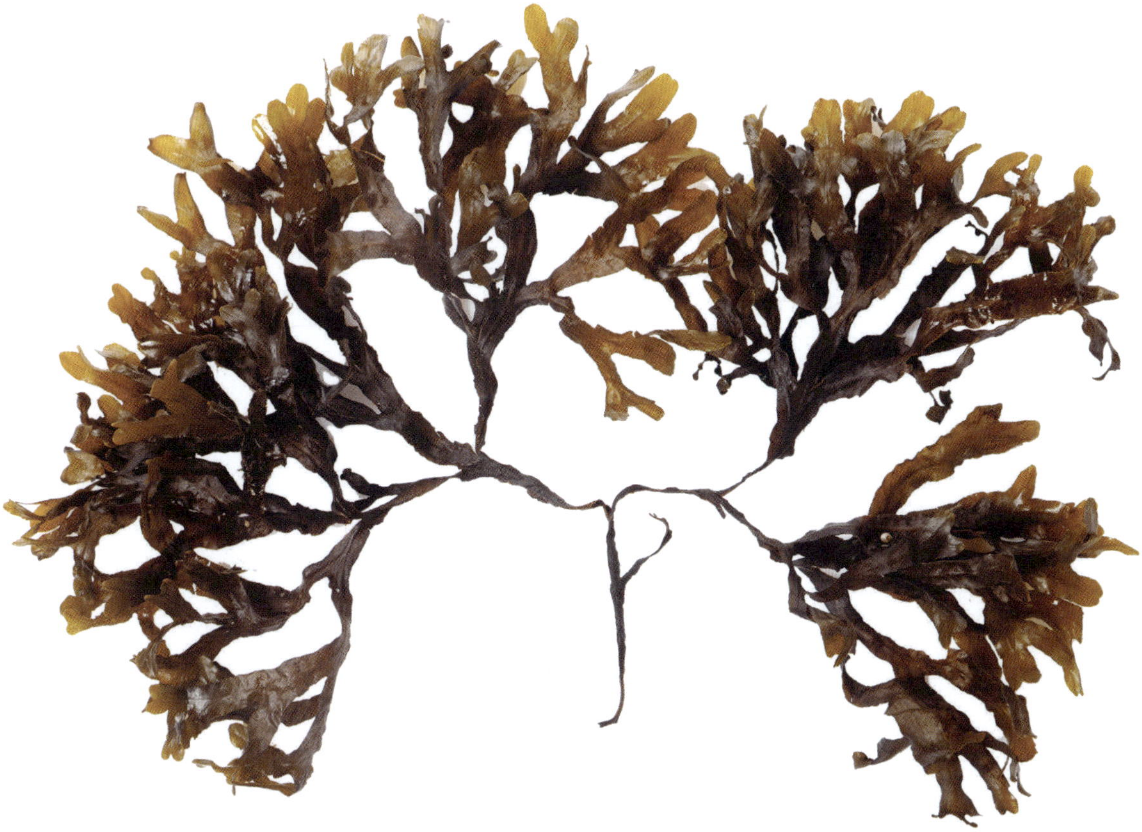

Undaria pinnatifida

Japanese seaweed, specifically wakame, contains several nutrients that can promote deeper sleep. For instance, wakame is a good source of glycine. This amino acid acts as a neurotransmitter and can improve sleep quality by promoting relaxation and reducing muscle spasms. Additionally, wakame is rich in magnesium, a mineral that is vital in regulating the body's sleep-wake cycle and increasing sleep efficiency. Moreover, the omega-3 fatty acids in wakame have been linked to better sleep quality and reduced symptoms of sleep disorders.

Wellbeing challenge: LIGHT SLEEP
Support ingredient: WAKAME

AVOCADO

The avocado is a remarkable fruit, with a unique shape and texture that make it instantly recognizable. With its smooth and creamy flesh, avocado has become a popular ingredient in beauty products and skincare practices thanks to its nourishing and hydrating properties. This fruit has taken the beauty world by storm, from face masks to hair treatments, proving that its benefits extend beyond delightful toast topping.

The avocado, scientifically known as *Persea americana*, is native to Central America but is now cultivated worldwide. This pear-shaped fruit contains heart-healthy monounsaturated fats, vitamins and minerals. Its creamy texture makes it a popular ingredient in various dishes, from guacamole to avocado toast. But beyond the kitchen, the avocado has numerous uses. Its oil is a natural moisturizer often used in skincare products, and the fruit is a popular ingredient in DIY hair masks (just ask your favourite beauty influencer). Moreover, its large seed creates natural dyes, and its wood is highly valued for its durability and decorative properties.

HISTORY

Legend has it that the avocado was once called the 'testicle fruit' by the Aztecs, who believed its shape and properties symbolized fertility and vitality. Later, Spanish explorers brought avocado to Europe and introduced it to other parts of the world. It was in the twentieth century that avocados gained popularity in the United States and became a staple ingredient in Mexican cuisine. Today, avocados are widely enjoyed worldwide, and their versatility and health benefits continue to make them a favourite fruit for many.

Persea americana

Avocado oil is rich in vitamins, antioxidants and fatty acids, making it a trusted choice for improving the appearance of dull skin. Its high oleic acid content helps to hydrate and nourish the skin, while its anti-inflammatory properties can help reduce redness and irritation. Avocado oil also contains lutein and zeaxanthin, which can help protect the skin from UV damage. When applied topically, avocado oil can help to improve skin elasticity, reduce the appearance of fine lines and wrinkles, and leave the skin looking soft and radiant. Its moisturizing properties make it an ideal ingredient in anatomē's skincare formulations, such as facial oils and moisturizers.

Wellbeing challenge: DULL, DRY SKIN
Support ingredient: AVOCADO

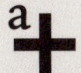

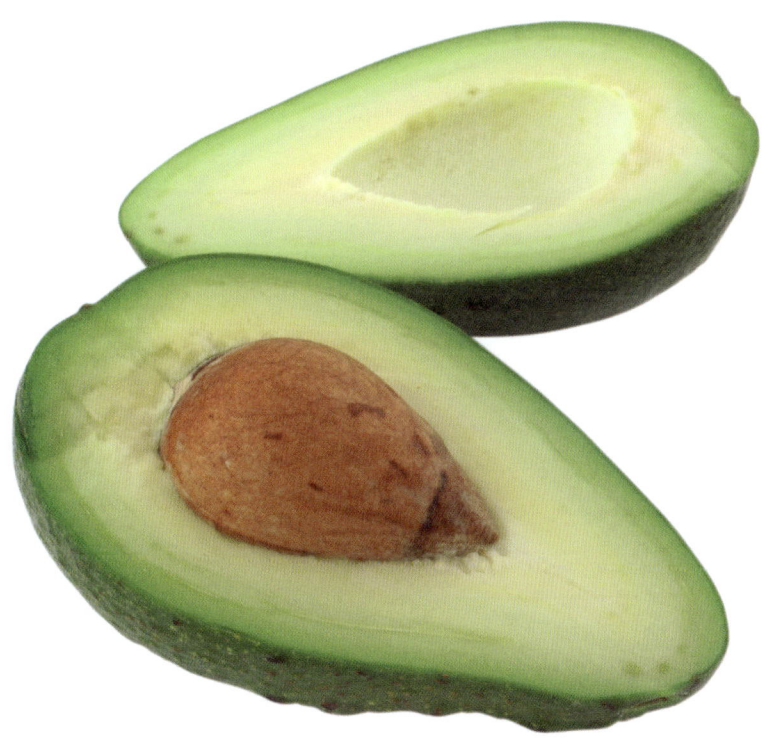

HERO BOTANICALS

GRAPE SEED

Grapes, those versatile orbs of juicy sweetness, are often enjoyed seedless, but have you ever stopped to appreciate the seeds? Like tiny gems, they gleam amidst the flesh, offering a glimpse into the fruit's past and future. Yes, we spit them out, but in the right hands, those humble seeds can be a source of endless possibilities, from crafting to skincare.

Despite their numerous health benefits, grape seeds, or *Vitis vinifera* seeds, are often overlooked. These tiny seeds are rich in antioxidants, including proanthocyanidins, which are known to promote cardiovascular health and reduce inflammation. Grape seed oil is used in dietary supplements and skincare products for its antioxidant properties. In cooking, this oil is popular due to its high smoke point and neutral taste. We can grind grape seeds – turning them into flour for baking, or use them as a natural dye. In addition to their culinary and medicinal uses, grape seeds are a popular craft material, used from jewellery to home decor.

HISTORY

Grape seeds have featured as a staple ingredient since ancient times. The earliest evidence of their use dates to the ancient Egyptians, who used grape seeds in their burial rituals. In medieval Europe, grape seeds were used to make oil and vinegar. In the twentieth century, grape seed extract gained popularity for its antioxidant properties. Today, grape seeds are a valuable resource for their culinary and medicinal uses. From ancient times to the modern day, grape seeds have stood the test of time as a versatile and beneficial ingredient.

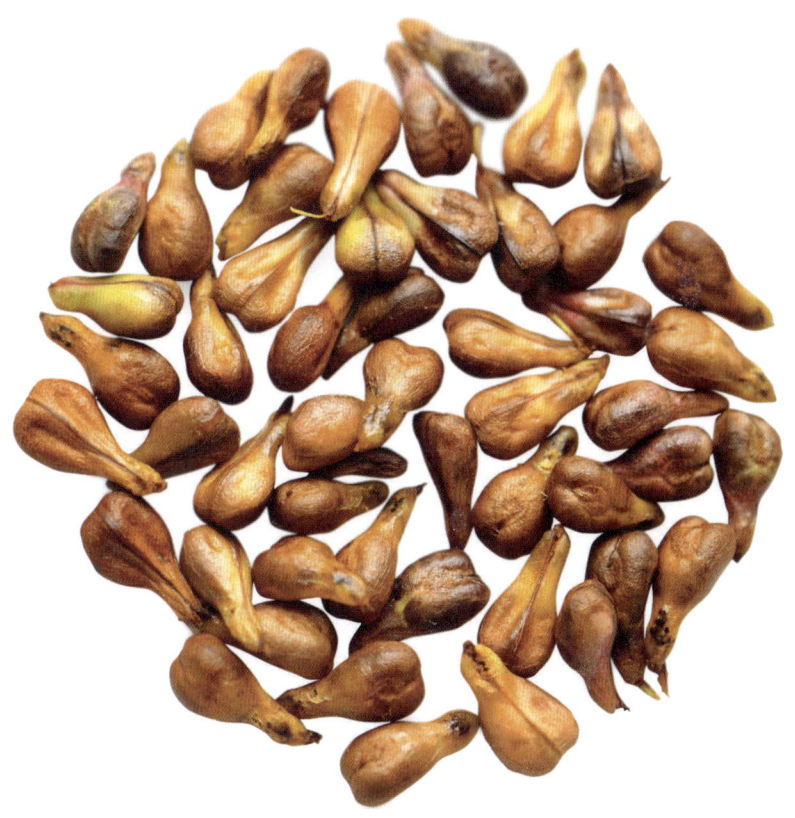

Vitis vinifera

Grape seed oil is a popular skincare ingredient and in many of anatomē's skin formulations, due to its numerous benefits. It is high in linoleic acid, which helps to strengthen the skin barrier and prevent moisture loss, making it especially beneficial for those with dry or sensitive skin. Grape seed oil is also rich in antioxidants, which help to protect the skin from damage caused by free radicals and UV rays. When applied topically, grape seed oil can help to improve the appearance of dull skin, reduce the appearance of fine lines and wrinkles, and even out skin tone. Its non-comedogenic properties make it an excellent choice for those with acne-prone skin.

Wellbeing challenge: ACNE-PRONE SKIN
Support ingredient: GRAPE SEED

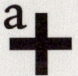

ALOE VERA

Aloe vera, the succulent plant known for its healing properties, has been used for centuries for its medicinal benefits. With its long, spiky leaves and gel-filled interior, it's easy to see why this plant has captured the imagination of many. Whether you've used it to soothe a sunburn or admired its unique aesthetic, aloe vera is a plant that has earned its place in our homes and hearts.

Aloe vera, also known as *Aloe Barbadensis*, is a succulent plant from North Africa. It is prized for its medicinal properties, containing antibacterial and anti-inflammatory compounds. The gel-like substance extracted from the plant's leaves soothes skin irritations and promotes wound healing. In addition to its topical uses, aloe vera can also be consumed for its potential health benefits, such as aiding in digestion and promoting healthy skin from within. This versatile plant has also found its way into various cosmetics and personal care products due to its moisturizing and anti-ageing properties.

HISTORY

Throughout history, this plant has been used for medicinal purposes by different cultures, including the ancient Egyptians, who called it the 'plant of immortality'. Legend has it that Alexander the Great used aloe vera to heal his soldiers' wounds. Its healing properties were also recognized by the Greeks and Romans, who used it to treat burns, wounds and other skin conditions.

Aloe Barbadensis

Aloe vera is recognized for its numerous benefits in skin care. The gel extracted from the aloe vera plant leaves contains vitamins, minerals and antioxidants that help moisturize and soothe the skin. When applied topically, the gel acts as a natural moisturizer, penetrating the skin to provide hydration without leaving a greasy residue. Aloe vera also contains anti-inflammatory properties, making it an ideal ingredient for reducing redness and irritation. Additionally, aloe vera promotes collagen production, which can help improve the skin's elasticity and firmness.

Wellbeing challenge: SKIN REDNESS
Support ingredient: ALOE VERA

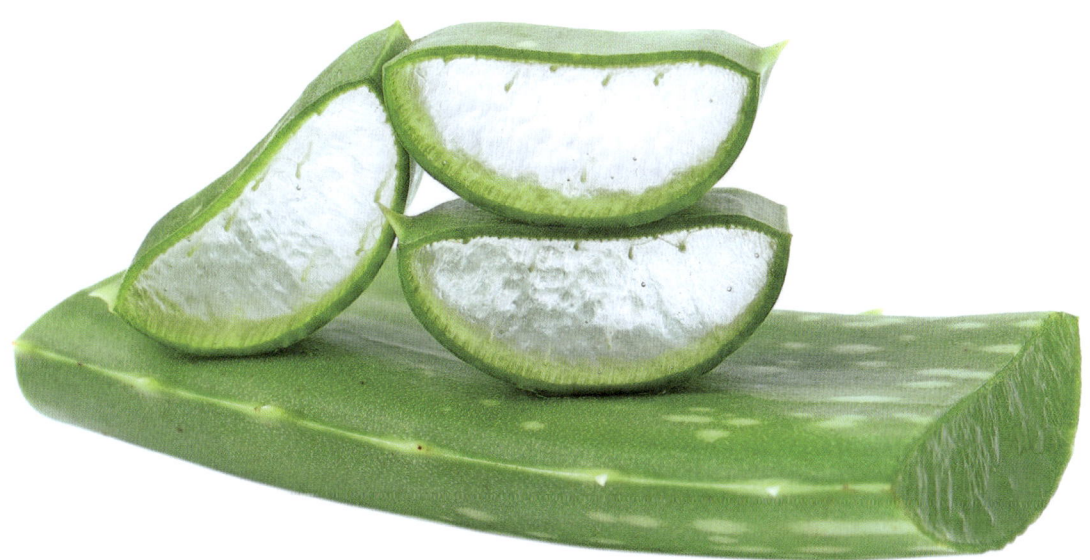

JOJOBA

Imagine a vast desert landscape with scorching sun and arid winds. Yet amidst the harsh environment, a resilient plant thrives – the jojoba. Its small, oval-shaped fruits are a sight to behold, with a striking green hue and a velvety texture. Native to North America, jojoba has been used for centuries by indigenous communities for its nourishing properties. Today, jojoba reigns in the beauty industry for its ability to moisturize and protect the skin, hair and nails.

Jojoba oil, derived from the seeds of the *Simmondsia chinensis* plant, is a versatile and widely used oil in skincare and haircare products. It has a unique chemical structure, similar to human sebum, that allows it to absorb quickly and deeply into the skin. Jojoba oil is rich in antioxidants, vitamins and minerals that can help improve the texture and appearance of the skin, reduce inflammation and promote healthy hair growth. It is commonly used in massage oils, facial serums and conditioners, as well as in cooking and as a carrier oil for essential oils.

HISTORY

Jojoba oil has a relatively short history compared to many other plant-based oils. It was first discovered in the early eighteenth century by Native Americans, who used the oil for its medicinal and cosmetic properties. In the 1970s, Jojoba oil gained popularity in the cosmetic industry as a natural and effective ingredient in skincare products. Its unique chemical properties and texture make it versatile in many products, from makeup removers to hair conditioners.

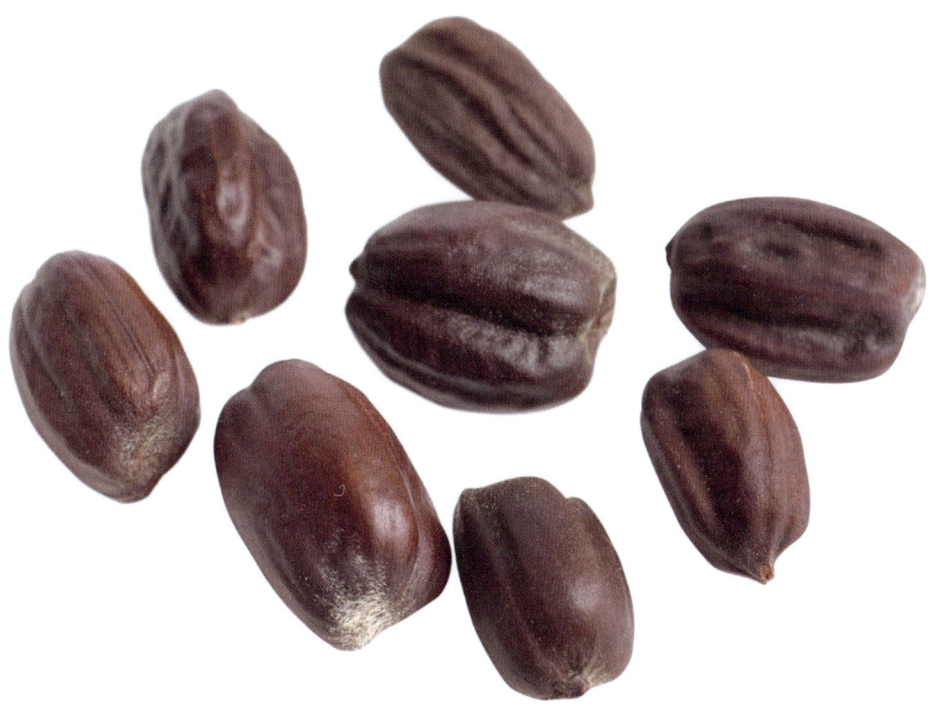

Simmondsia chinensis

Jojoba oil is a light golden liquid with a non-greasy texture, rich in vitamin E, antioxidants and essential fatty acids. It has exceptional emollient properties that help to retain moisture in the skin and improve its elasticity, making it an excellent option for dry skin – and a trusted ingredient in our skincare formulations. It is also anti-inflammatory and antibacterial, making it an effective treatment for acne-prone skin. It can also soothe sunburns and reduce the appearance of fine lines and wrinkles.

Wellbeing challenge: DRY SKIN
Support ingredient: JOJOBA

HIMALAYAN SALT

Not a botanical (the only exception to the rule in this book), but a mineral ingredient with powerful properties, Himalayan salt, like a sparkling crystal from a hidden treasure trove, carries the essence of ancient mountains. Its delicate blush hues and jagged edges evoke a sense of wonder as if you are holding a piece of the majestic Himalayas.

Himalayan salt, revered for its pink colour and unique mineral composition, originates from the Khewra Salt Mine in Pakistan. Crystal lamps made from it are believed to release negative ions, purifying the air. Himalayan salt, scientifically revered for its mineral-rich composition, offers numerous benefits when incorporated into baths. It contains essential minerals like magnesium, potassium and calcium. When dissolved in warm water, these minerals are absorbed through the skin, promoting relaxation and soothing tired muscles. And it has its place in the kitchen: it draws admirers who appreciate its natural origins and distinctive rosy hue, adding a touch of elegance (and a conversation point) to their culinary creations.

HISTORY

Himalayan salt boasts a rich history rooted in the majestic Himalayan mountains. It was formed over 250 million years ago, and its genesis lies in ancient oceans that evaporated, leaving behind vast salt deposits. For centuries, the Khewra Salt Mine has been its primary source, first discovered by the troops of Alexander the Great in 326 BC. This mineral treasure remained largely untapped until British colonial rule in India when a mine was developed.

Pink Halite

Himalayan salt baths can aid detoxification by drawing out impurities and reducing inflammation. When used in bath salts and scrubs, it promotes relaxation and exfoliation. It also has natural antimicrobial properties, which can assist in maintaining healthy skin. Additionally, the gentle exfoliating effect of Himalayan salt can leave the skin feeling soft, smooth and rejuvenated.

Wellbeing challenge: INFLAMMATION
Support ingredient: HIMALAYAN SALT

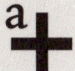

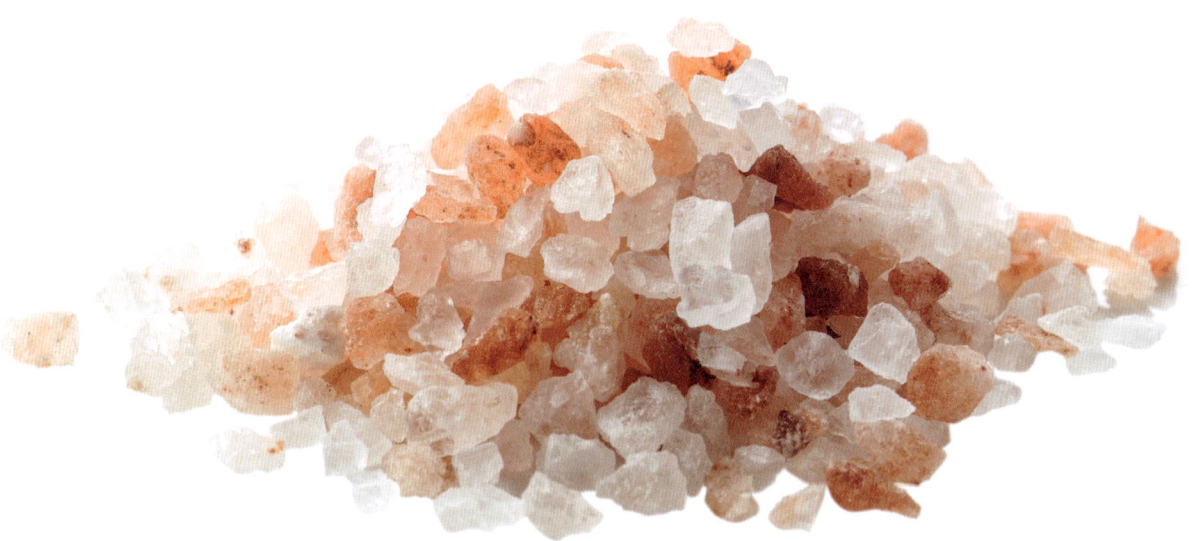

HERO BOTANICALS

ENGLISH PEPPERMINT

With its vibrant green leaves and strong, refreshing scent, English peppermint is like a cool breeze on a hot summer day. Its aroma awakens the senses and invigorates the mind, making it a popular choice for teas and aromatherapy. When crushed between the fingers, its leaves release a fragrance that can transport us to a peaceful English garden, surrounded by blooming flowers and buzzing bees.

Scientifically known as *Mentha piperita*, this type of peppermint originates from the UK and is a hybrid of watermint and spearmint – extracted from the leaves and stems of the plant. Its main component, menthol, has a cooling effect on the skin and can help to soothe sore muscles. Peppermint oil is often used in cooking to add a fresh, minty flavour to desserts and drinks. It is also commonly used in aromatherapy and personal care products such as toothpaste, shampoos and soaps.

HISTORY

English peppermint oil's history goes back to ancient times and it was used by the Greeks, Romans and Egyptians for medicinal purposes. It was cultivated in England since the 1700s, and it quickly became one of the most popular herbs used in medicine, culinary arts and perfumery. During World War II, peppermint oil was also used to treat headaches and fatigue.

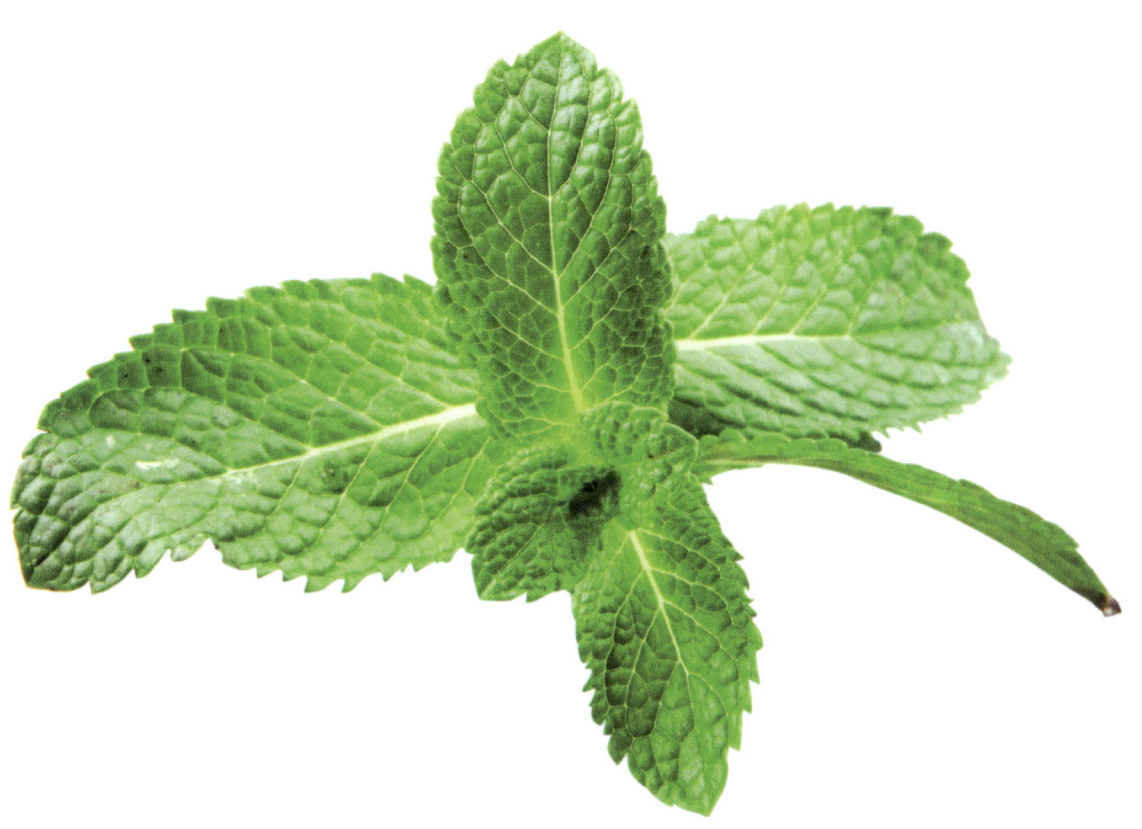

Mentha piperita

English peppermint oil has been used for centuries for its therapeutic benefits, particularly boosting energy levels and protecting against harmful pathogens – two benefits we harness in our formulations. Peppermint oil contains menthol, which increases alertness and enhances mental focus. It also has antimicrobial properties that can help protect against infections caused by bacteria, viruses and fungi. When applied topically, peppermint oil can provide a cooling sensation and help relieve sore muscles and joint pain. Overall, English peppermint oil is a versatile and effective essential oil with benefits for physical and mental wellbeing.

Wellbeing challenge: LOW ENERGY
Support ingredient: ENGLISH PEPPERMINT

NEROLI

Neroli, a delicate and intoxicating scent, is like a gentle breeze carrying the sweetest scent of blooming orange blossoms through the air, making you want to close your eyes and breathe deeply. A single drop can transport you to the Mediterranean, where the sun warms your skin and the sea sparkles in the distance.

Neroli is an essential oil extracted from the flowers of bitter orange trees, known scientifically as *Citrus aurantium*. It originates from the Middle East, but we can find it in various parts of the world today. This versatile oil has a sweet and floral aroma commonly used in perfumes, cosmetics and aromatherapy. It's also a popular ingredient in personal care and therapeutic products – including anatomē's formulations. It has anti-inflammatory and antiseptic properties, benefiting its use in skincare. But that's not all: neroli oil reduces anxiety, promotes relaxation and alleviates digestive problems.

HISTORY

Legend has it that neroli was named after an Italian princess who loved the scent of bitter orange blossom, from which the oil is extracted. The Moors brought bitter orange trees to Spain, where the oil became popular during the Renaissance. Today, neroli is still cherished for its versatile nature and enchanting aroma, making it a beloved ingredient in the world of natural beauty and wellness.

Citrus aurantium

Neroli oil's invigorating scent has been shown to have a positive effect on mood and energy levels. The oil contains chemical compounds such as linalool and limonene that have stimulating and energizing properties. When used in aromatherapy, neroli oil can help improve focus, concentration and productivity. Additionally, it is believed to have antioxidant properties that may protect skin from damage caused by free radicals. It can be diluted with a carrier oil and applied topically or diffused in a room to promote a sense of vitality and alertness.

Wellbeing challenge: LOW FOCUS
Support ingredient: NEROLI

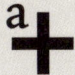

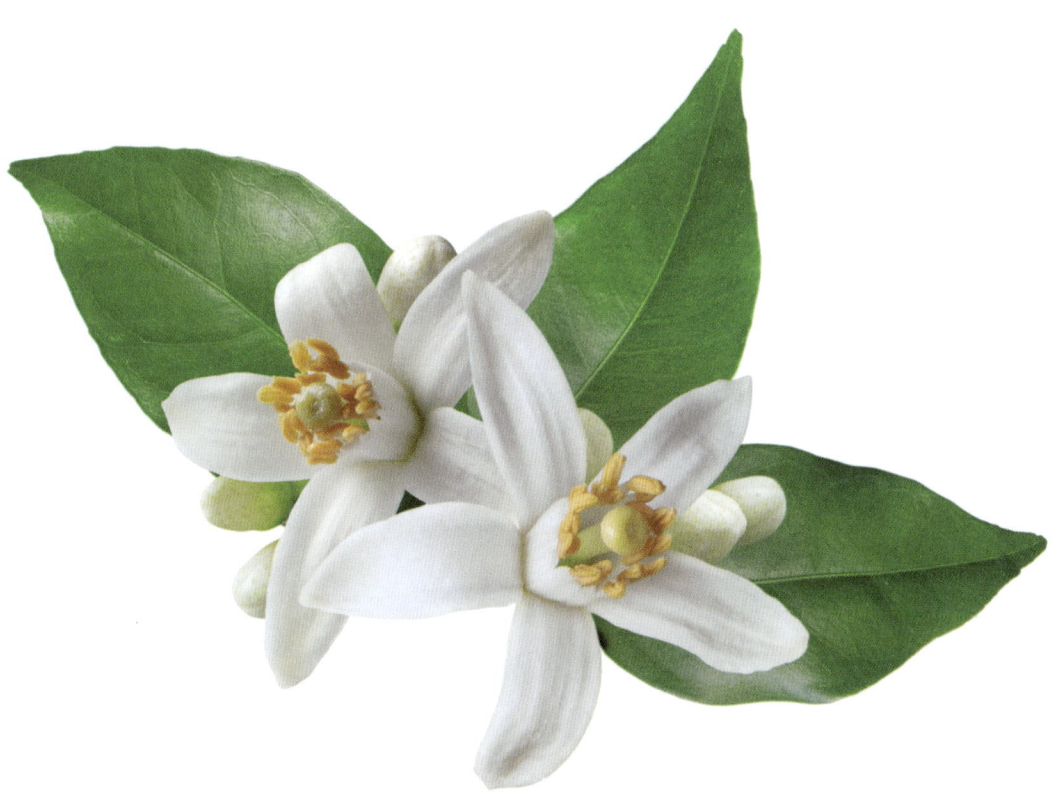

HERO BOTANICALS

EUCALYPTUS

The crisp, refreshing scent of eucalyptus takes us to Australia's cool, misty forests. This potent plant has been a staple of traditional medicine for centuries, renowned for its ability to invigorate the senses and promote respiratory health. At anatomē, we believe in the power of eucalyptus, whether we're looking to clear our sinuses or transport ourselves to a tranquil oasis.

Eucalyptus oil, also known as 'gum tree oil', comes from the leaves of the eucalyptus tree. Its scientific name is *Eucalyptus globulus*. This tree is native to Australia, but we can find it in many other parts of the world today. Eucalyptus oil has a strong, fresh, minty aroma and is widely used in aromatherapy for its refreshing and energizing properties. It's also known for its antibacterial, antifungal and anti-inflammatory properties. In addition to aromatherapy, eucalyptus oil is the star ingredient in products such as cough drops, chest rubs and is also used as a natural insect repellent, which take us back to childhood holidays.

HISTORY

Eucalyptus trees have a long history in their native Australia, where indigenous peoples have used the leaves for medicinal purposes for thousands of years. Only in the nineteenth century did eucalyptus oil begin to be extracted and used in Western medicine. During World War I, this oil was in high demand for its antiseptic properties, and the eucalyptus industry boomed.

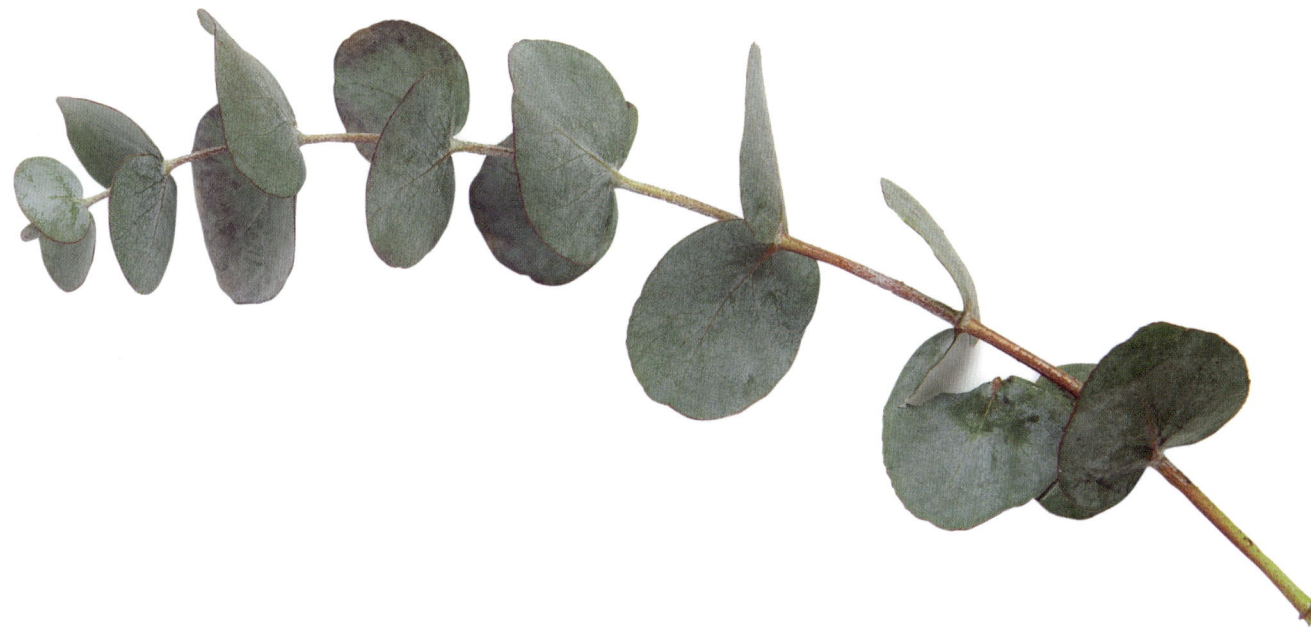

Eucalyptus globulus

Eucalyptus oil is known for its strong, refreshing scent and is commonly used in aromatherapy. It has antiseptic, antibacterial and antiviral properties, making it popular for promoting immunity and protection against illnesses. We can apply it topically on the skin or inhale it through steam to help clear the respiratory system. It also features as an ingredient in cleaning and disinfecting products for its powerful disinfectant properties.

Wellbeing challenge: WEAK IMMUNITY
Support ingredient: EUCALYPTUS

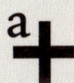

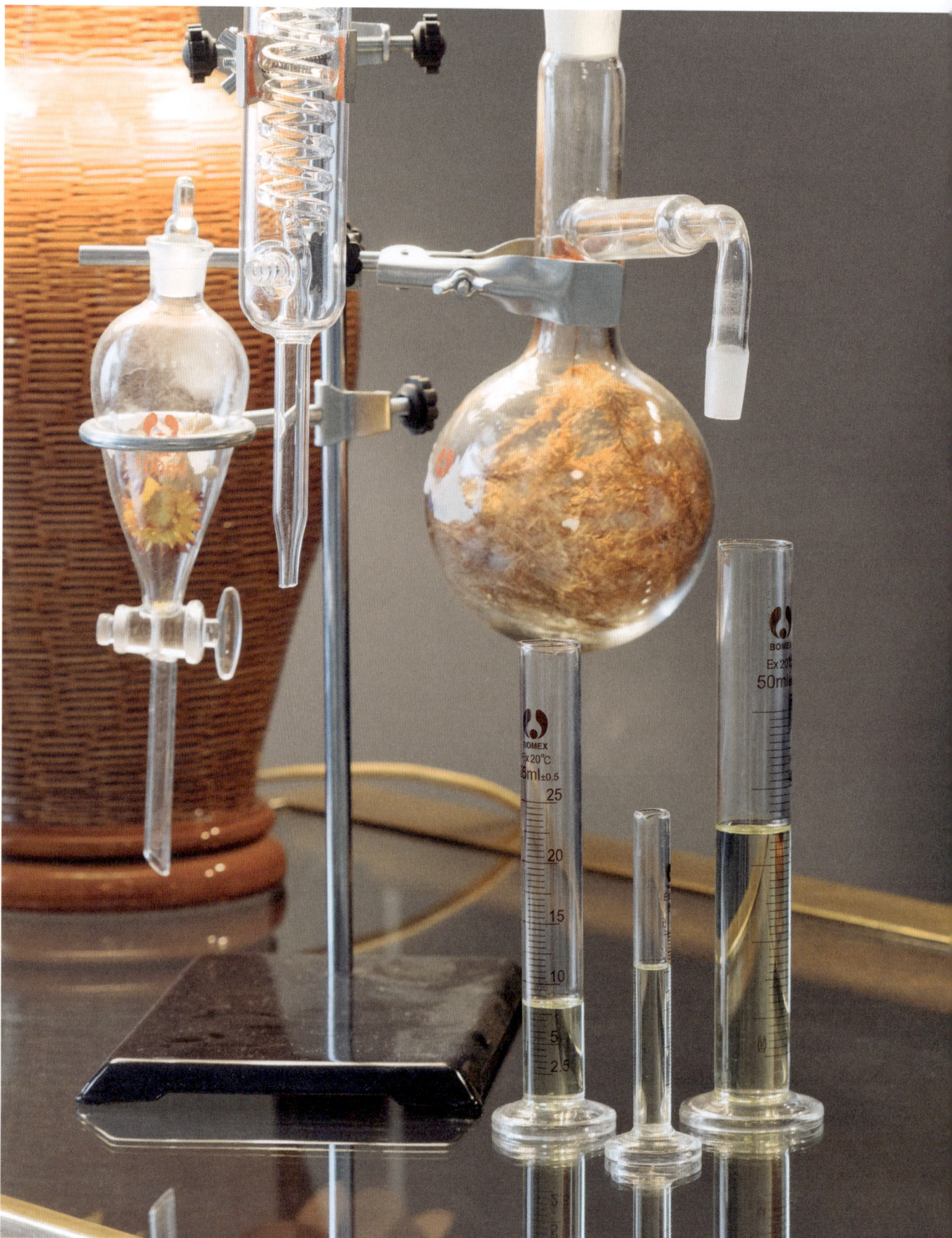

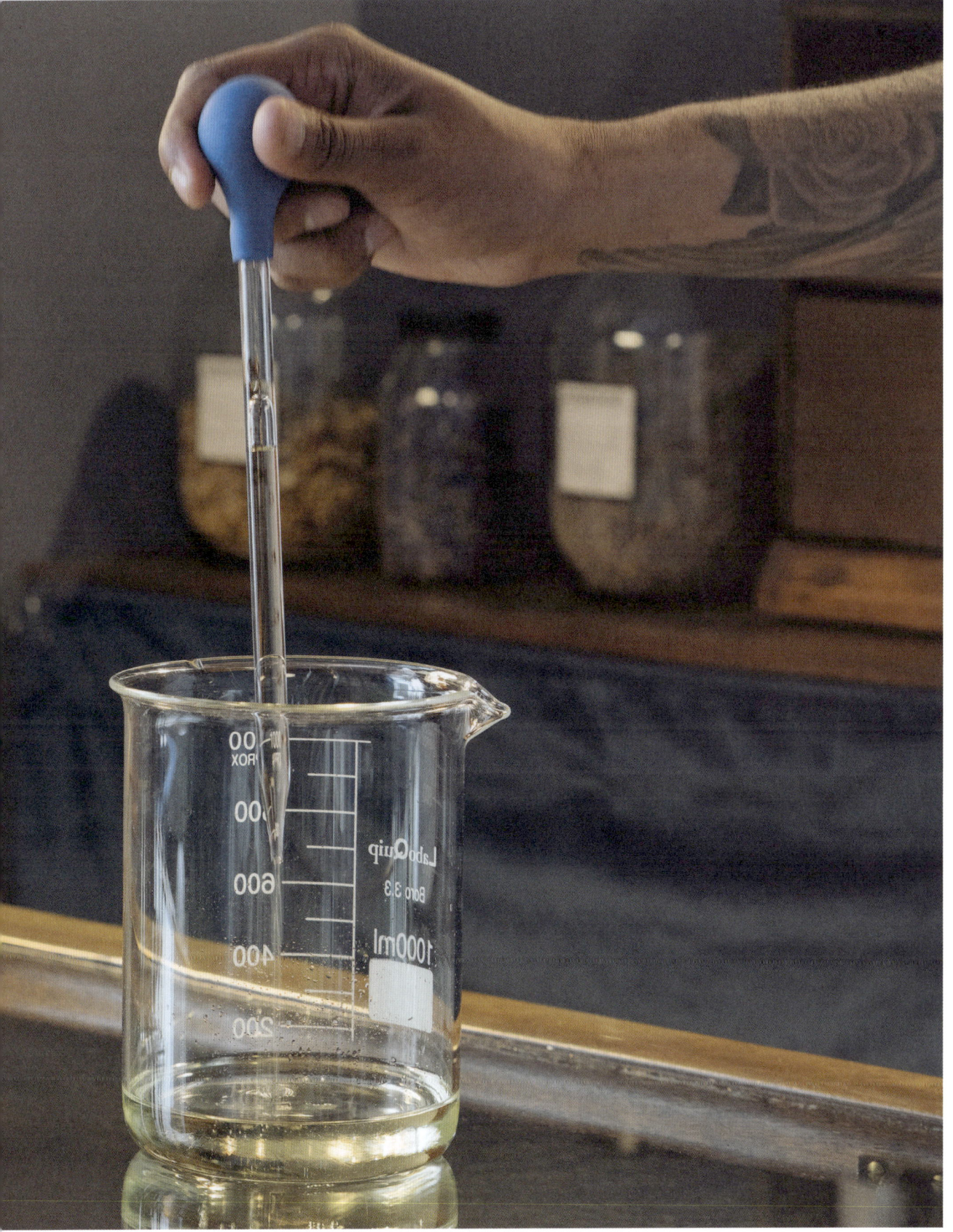

TEA TREE

Amidst the vast Australian bushland, a small shrub stands out for its powerful essence. With its vibrant leaves and white flowers, tea tree has long been treasured by indigenous communities for its healing properties. The potent oil extracted from its leaves has found its way into many modern homes, bringing a distinct herbal aroma and many benefits.

Tea tree oil is extracted from the leaves of the tea tree plant, native to Australia. It has a clear, fresh and camphor-like scent and properties, including antiseptic, antifungal and antibacterial. It's used to treat acne, wounds and insect bites and clears fungal infections such as dandruff and athlete's foot. In cooking, it is used to add flavour to certain dishes. Additionally, it is a common ingredient in homemade cleaning products due to its antimicrobial properties.

HISTORY

The indigenous people of Australia have long known about the benefits of the tea tree plant, and it has been used for centuries to treat infectious ailments. Captain James Cook, an English explorer, encountered the plant during his voyage to Australia and named it the 'tea tree' because he brewed a tea-like drink from its leaves. In the early 1900s, the oil extracted from this plant was found to have powerful antibacterial properties, and it became a popular treatment for wounds during World War II. Tea tree oil is used in various household and skincare products today for its antibacterial and antifungal properties.

Melaleuca alternifolia

Tea tree oil features in anatomē's essential oil blends for different purposes. It has potent antiseptic and anti-inflammatory properties, making it a popular ingredient for treating acne, eczema and other skin conditions. Tea tree oil is also known for boosting immunity and protecting against infections. When used topically, it can help to disinfect wounds and promote healing. Additionally, this oil has a refreshing and invigorating scent, making it a popular choice for aromatherapy to help energize the mind and body.

Wellbeing challenge: SKIN ISSUES
Support ingredient: TEA TREE

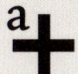

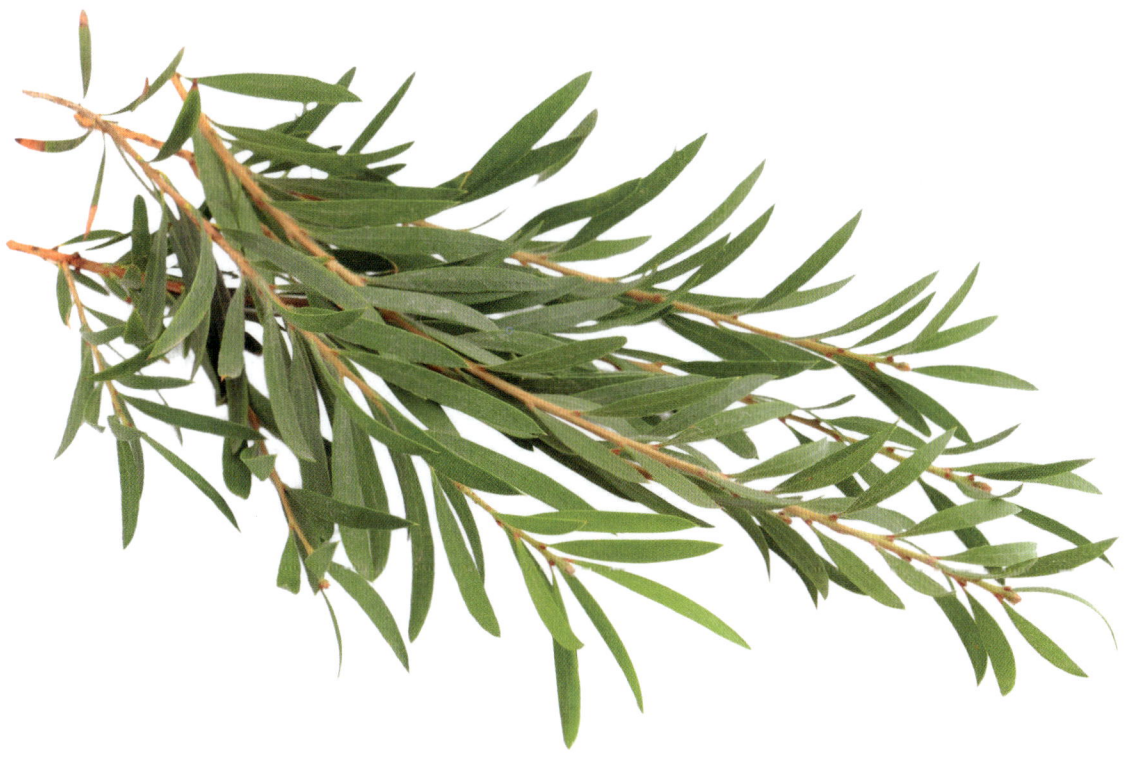

HERO BOTANICALS

CAMPHOR

Have you ever felt that tingly, refreshing sensation after using a vapour rub? That's thanks to the powerful ingredient of camphor. This natural compound has been used for centuries to invigorate the senses and awaken the mind. From its cool, crisp scent to its revitalizing properties, camphor is the perfect pick-me-up for sluggish mornings or mid-afternoon slumps.

Camphor oil is derived from the camphor tree, known scientifically as *Cinnamomum camphora*, and has been used for its medicinal properties for centuries. It has a distinct, fresh and invigorating scent commonly used in aromatherapy to enhance focus and promote respiratory health. Camphor oil has analgesic, antifungal and antiseptic properties, making it a popular ingredient in medicinal and cosmetic products. Other common uses include as an insect repellent, a pain reliever for sore muscles and joints and a component in cough and cold remedies.

HISTORY

Camphor's history dates back to ancient China and Japan, where it was used in medicinal and spiritual practices. Its name is derived from the Sanskrit word *karpura*, and it was traded along the Silk Road for its aromatic and medicinal properties. In Europe, it was used in embalming and later in medicine. During World War I, camphor made part of the ingredients list to produce explosives. This ingredient is still used in traditional medicine and modern products such as topical ointments, insect repellents and cleaning products.

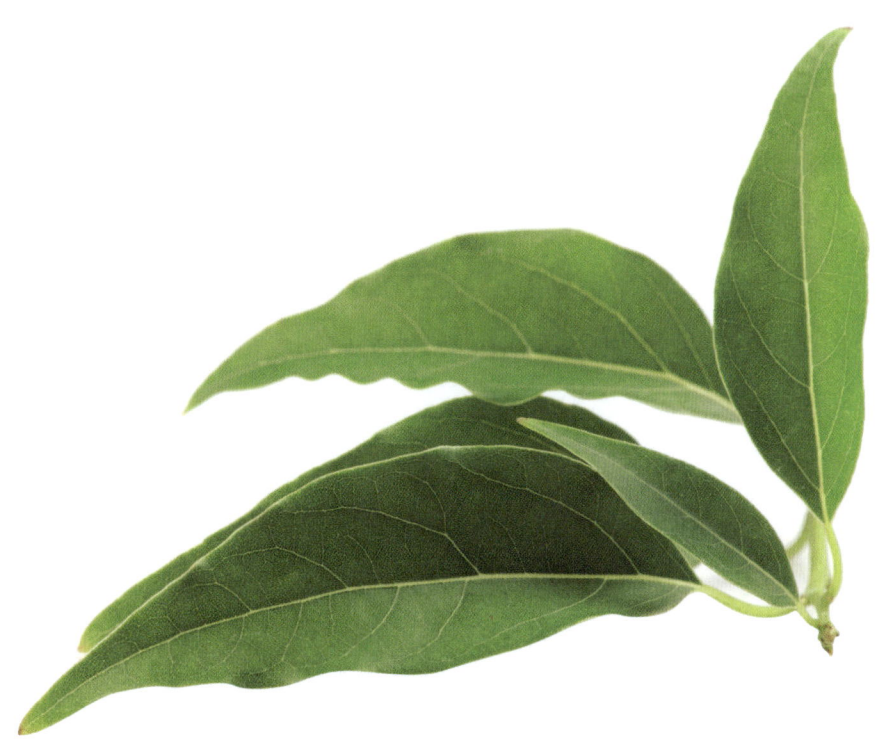

Cinnamomum camphora

Camphor oil is rich in antiseptic compounds, including camphor, terpene and safrole, which give it a fresh, minty aroma. It can help relieve pain, itching and irritation when used topically due to its anti-inflammatory properties. It is also a potent antiseptic, making it an effective treatment for minor cuts and wounds. Breathing this oil during a practice has been shown to boost immunity and help our self-expression, opening our airways and ourselves.

Wellbeing challenge: MINOR WOUNDS
Support ingredient: CAMPHOR

LION'S MANE

Imagine a lion with a magnificent, flowing mane. Now picture that same lion with a brain the size of a human's. That's the essence of lion's mane, a mushroom with a regal name and impressive cognitive benefits. No, it won't make you roar like a lion, but it might just give your brain the royal treatment it deserves.

Scientifically known as *Hericium erinaceus*, lion's mane is an edible mushroom native to Asia, Europe and North America. This unique-looking mushroom has long, white, hair-like spines that resemble a lion's mane, hence its name. It has been traditionally used in Chinese medicine for its potential health benefits, which include boosting cognitive function, improving heart health and supporting the immune system. Lion's mane is also commonly used in culinary dishes, with its meaty texture and nutty flavour, making it a popular meat substitute for vegetarian and vegan dishes. This miracle ingredient also has anti-inflammatory and antioxidant properties.

HISTORY

Lion's mane has been used in traditional Chinese medicine for centuries. Legend has it that a Taoist monk was wandering through the forest when he stumbled upon a patch of mushrooms growing on a dead tree. Upon closer inspection, the monk noticed that the mushrooms resembled a lion's mane and decided to try them. He felt invigorated and believed that the mushroom had powerful medicinal properties. From then on, lion's mane has been valuable in Chinese culture.

Hericium erinaceus

Lion's mane is widely used for its cognitive benefits. It contains compounds such as erinacines and hericenones known to stimulate nerve growth factors, promoting the growth and regeneration of brain cells. Studies have shown that lion's mane can improve cognitive function, memory and focus, making it a popular natural nootropic. Its antioxidant and anti-inflammatory properties make it beneficial for overall brain health. It can be consumed in supplement form or added to dishes for its nutty flavour and health benefits and be used to support the immune system, reduce anxiety and depression and alleviate symptoms of neuropathy.

Wellbeing challenge: FOGGY BRAIN
Support ingredient: LION'S MANE

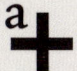

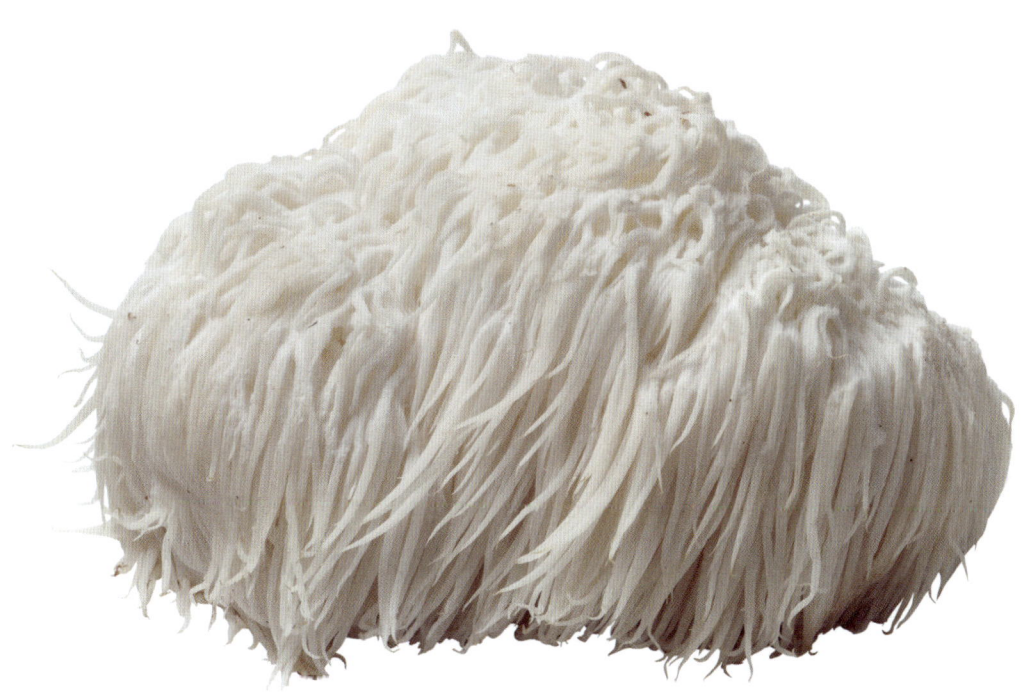

HERO BOTANICALS

BLACK PEPPER

Take a stroll through a bustling spice market, where the air is filled with the warm aroma of black pepper. The sound of vendors haggling and the vibrant colours of the spices create an atmosphere of excitement and adventure. Black pepper stands out among the many spices with its iconic aroma and rich history.

Black pepper, scientifically known as *Piper nigrum*, is a flowering vine that is native to southern India but is now grown in tropical regions worldwide. The small, dried fruit of the plant, commonly known as peppercorns, is a popular spice used in cuisines around the world. In addition to its culinary uses, black pepper also possesses medicinal properties, including anti-inflammatory and antioxidant effects. It is used in traditional medicine to treat ailments such as digestive issues and respiratory problems. Black pepper essential oil is also used in aromatherapy to alleviate stress and anxiety.

HISTORY

Black pepper has been used in cooking and medicine for thousands of years. It was highly valued in ancient times and was even used as a currency in some parts of the world. During the Middle Ages, black pepper was so valuable that it was sometimes used to pay rent and taxes. It played an important role in the spice trade, which was a major driver of global exploration and trade. Today, it is still one of the most widely used spices in the world and has a rich history and cultural significance.

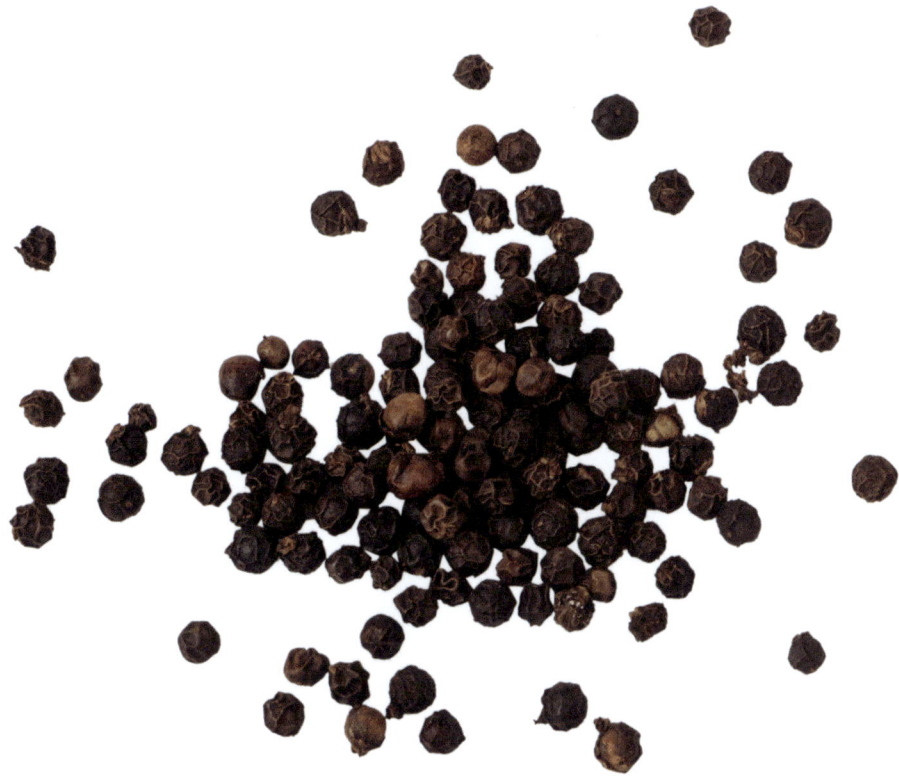

Piper nigrum

Black pepper essential oil – present in our focus formulations – is extracted from the dried fruit of the black pepper plant. It is a rich source of monoterpenes and sesquiterpenes, such as beta-caryophyllene, which contribute to its therapeutic benefits. When used aromatically, black pepper oil improves mood and enhances mental clarity and concentration. It also has stimulating and energizing properties, making it useful for combatting fatigue and increasing motivation and focus. The oil can be used topically to soothe muscle discomfort and promote healthy circulation. Its warming and invigorating qualities make it a popular addition to massage blends.

Wellbeing challenge: FATIGUE
Support ingredient: BLACK PEPPER

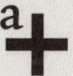

GINSENG

Have you ever wished you could bottle up the feeling you get after a great workout or a refreshing hike in nature? The ancient Chinese may have found the next best thing: ginseng. This root has been used for centuries to boost energy and vitality, and it's still a popular natural remedy today.

Ginseng is a plant with medicinal properties widely used in traditional Chinese medicine. The scientific name for ginseng is *Panax ginseng*, and it originates from Asia and North America. Ginseng is known to have antioxidant and anti-inflammatory properties, as well as benefits for mental health, such as improving focus, memory and reducing stress. Besides being used as a dietary supplement, ginseng can also be used in cooking, especially in Korean cuisine, where it is used in soups and other dishes. Ginseng has also been used topically for its potential benefits in skin health.

HISTORY

Legend has it that thousands of years ago, a Chinese emperor was exploring his kingdom when he came across a strange plant with a root that resembled a human form. Intrigued by its appearance, he tasted the root and found it to have a pleasantly stimulating effect. From then on, Chinese royalty highly sought after ginseng, which was believed to have medicinal properties that could enhance longevity and vitality. As trade routes expanded, ginseng found its way to other parts of the world and became one of the most valuable herbs in traditional medicine.

Panax ginseng

anatomē harnesses ginseng's benefits, applying it to many of its supplements. It contains ginsenosides: a group of bioactive compounds shown to reduce inflammation, improve cognitive function and boost immune system function.When used for hormonal support, ginseng may help regulate cortisol levels and improve symptoms of menopause. Additionally, ginseng may benefit gut health, increasing the growth of healthy gut bacteria and reducing inflammation in the gut.

Wellbeing challenge: LACK OF FOCUS
Support ingredient: GINSENG

a+

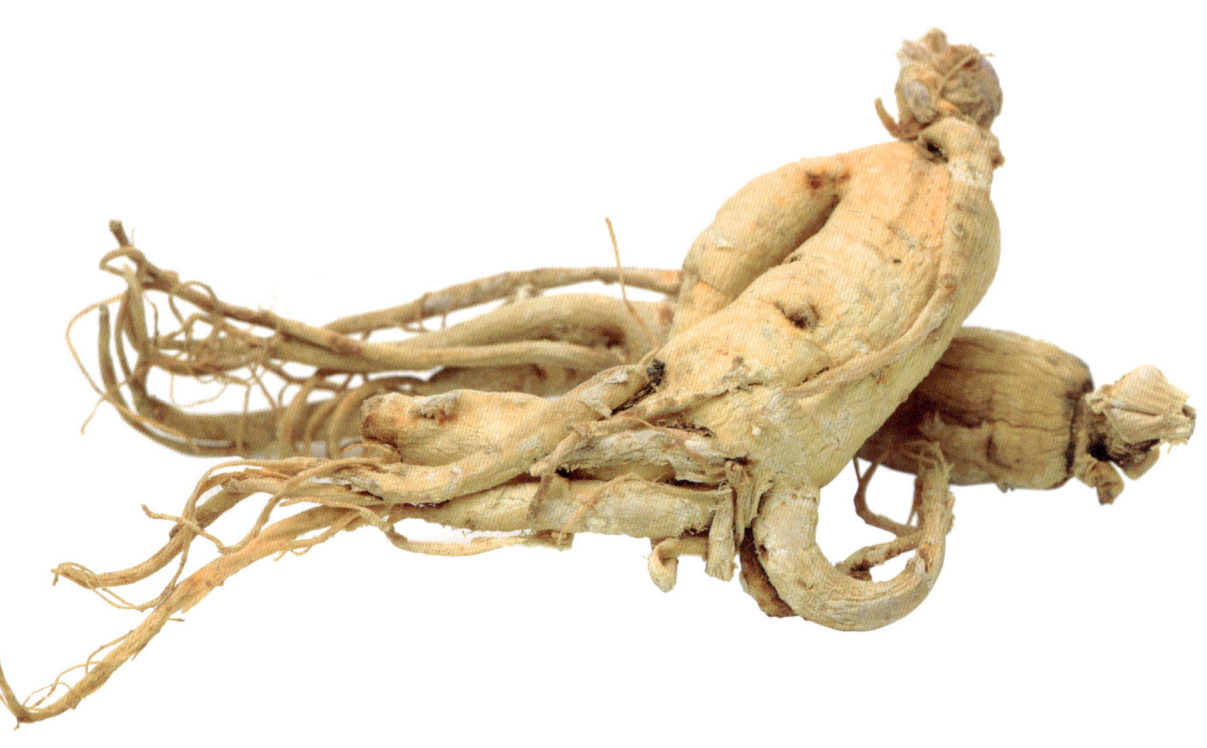

PRIMROSE

Primrose: this plant's name conjures images of delicate, velvety petals that glow in the soft light of a spring evening. As you close your eyes and breathe in their sweet fragrance, you can almost feel the gentle breeze on your face and the soft grass beneath your feet.

Scientifically known as *Oenothera biennis*, primrose is a biennial plant native to North and South America, although it can now be found growing all over the world. It is easily recognizable for its bright yellow flowers that bloom in the evening, giving off a sweet scent that attracts moths. The plant contains high amounts of essential fatty acids, such as gamma-linolenic acid, making it a popular herbal remedy for PMS symptoms, skin conditions and overall hormonal support. Primrose oil can be used in cooking and in skincare products, supplements and herbal remedies.

HISTORY

In the early seventeenth century, a botanist named John Goodyer came across a beautiful flower in the English countryside. He found that the plant's seeds would cure any 'violent paine in the head'. This discovery led to the plant being named 'primrose', derived from the Latin word for 'first rose', as it blooms early in the spring. The plant's medicinal properties were soon recognized, and it was used to treat a range of ailments, from respiratory issues to nervous disorders.

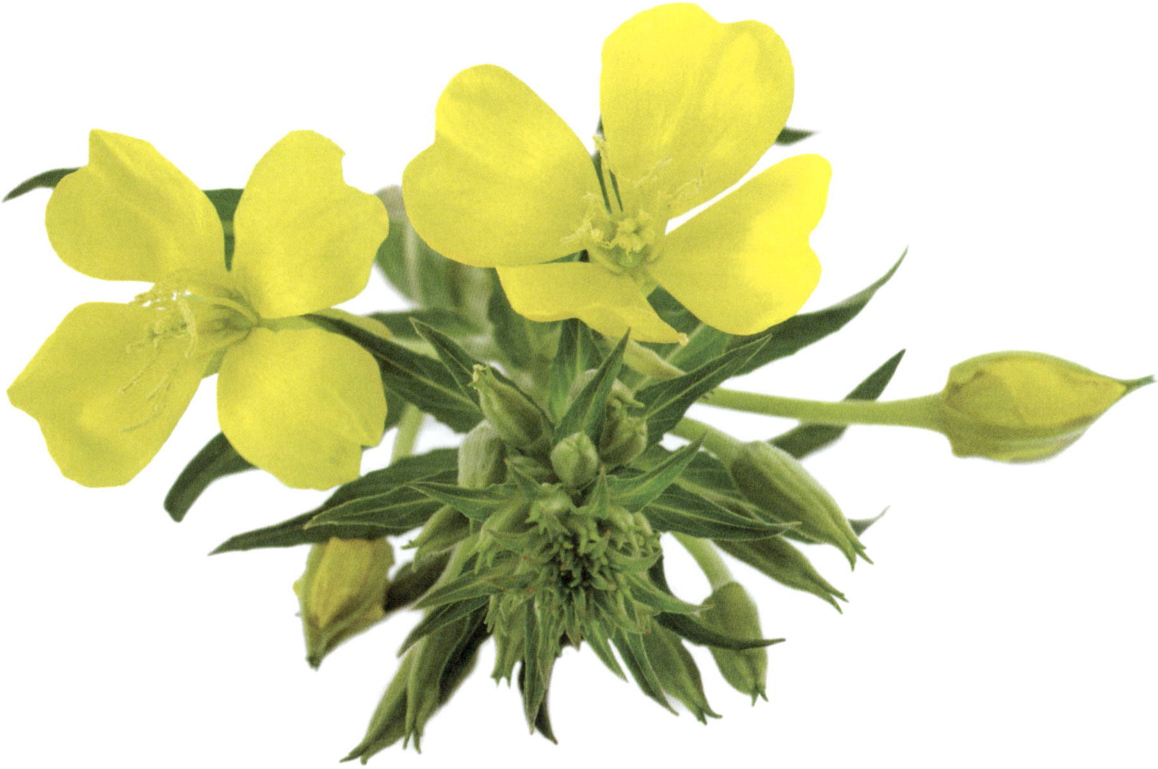

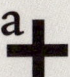

Oenothera biennis

Primrose oil is extracted from the evening primrose plant's seeds. It contains a high concentration of gamma-linolenic acid (GLA), an essential fatty acid that the body converts into prostaglandins. These hormone-like substances help regulate various bodily functions, including hormonal balance and inflammation. At anatomē, we apply it to our formulations supporting menopause, but primrose oil is also used to alleviate symptoms associated with premenstrual syndrome (PMS) and hormonal acne.

Wellbeing challenge: MENOPAUSE
Support ingredient: PRIMROSE

BLACK SPRUCE

The black spruce tree stands tall and proud, its branches reaching for the sky like a dancer's outstretched arms. Its scent is like a woodland symphony, filling the air with fresh pine and earthy musk harmony.

Black spruce, scientifically known as *Picea mariana*, is a species of evergreen tree native to Canada and parts of the United States. It is known for its fresh, woodsy scent and is often used in aromatherapy and as a natural remedy for various ailments. Its properties include being antiseptic, analgesic, and anti-inflammatory and its oil can be applied topically or diffused, promoting relaxation and reducing stress. The tree is also valued in the timber industry and has been used to construct everything from paper to canoes.

HISTORY

The story goes that the indigenous people of North America have long revered black spruce as a sacred tree with powerful medicinal properties. They used it to treat respiratory ailments, skin infections and even psychological distress. As European settlers arrived, they quickly recognized the tree's value for its solid and durable wood and began logging it extensively. Today, there are efforts to protect and restore black spruce forests, but the legacy of destruction remains, serving as a cautionary tale of humanity's impact on the natural world.

Piscea mariana

Black spruce essential oil contains high levels of chemical compounds including alpha-pinene, limonene and bornyl acetate. These compounds have antibacterial and anti-inflammatory properties, making black spruce oil beneficial for supporting gut health and the immune system. Additionally, black spruce oil has a grounding effect on the body and can help to balance hormonal imbalances. It can be diffused or applied topically when diluted in a carrier oil to reap its health benefits and is used in aromatherapy for its fresh, woody scent and centring effects.

Wellbeing challenge: UNGROUNDED MIND
Support ingredient: BLACK SPRUCE

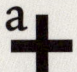

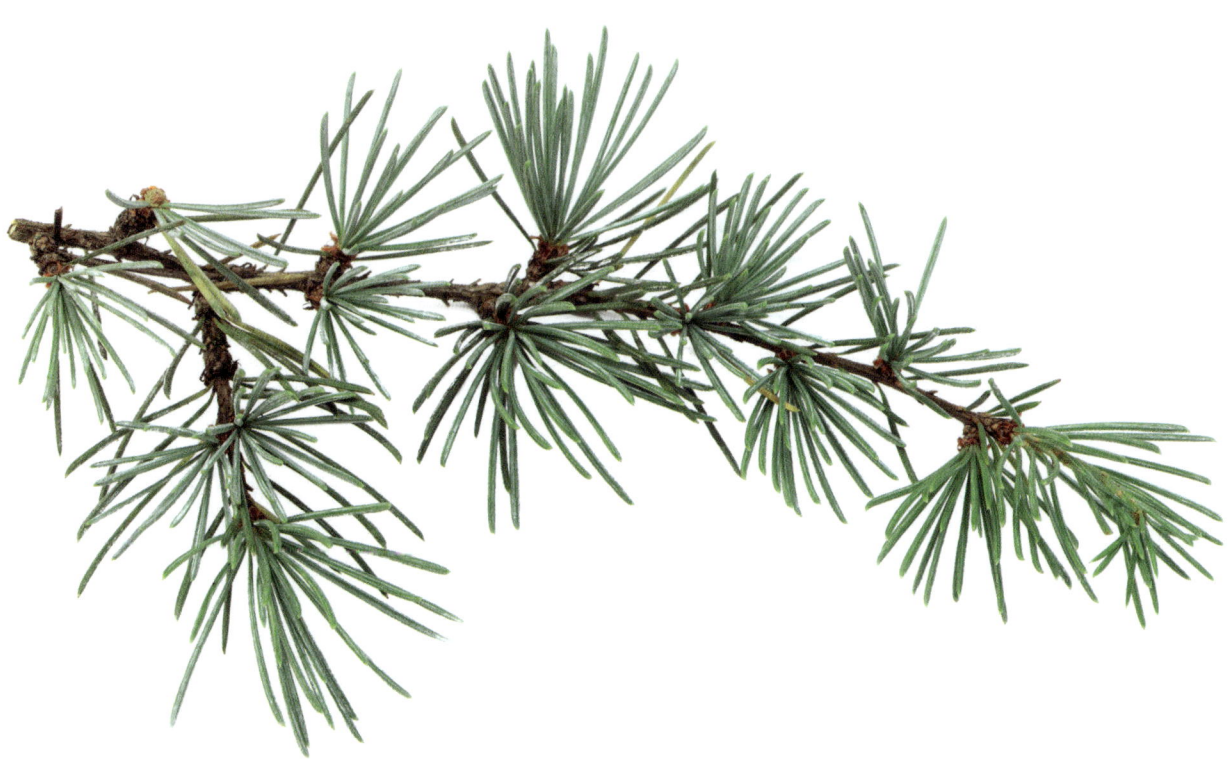

HERO BOTANICALS

ASHWAGANDHA

In ancient India, ashwagandha was thought to smell of horses, but don't let that fool you. This powerful herb has been used for centuries in Ayurvedic medicine to promote vitality and longevity.

Ashwagandha, also known as Indian ginseng or winter cherry, is native to India, the Middle East and parts of Africa. The plant has yellow flowers and produces red fruit, but its roots are used mostly for medicinal purposes. Ashwagandha is believed to have adaptogenic properties, which can help the body better cope with stress. It is also used for its anti-inflammatory and anti-anxiety effects, as well as for improving sleep, boosting energy and supporting the immune system. In cooking, ashwagandha is often used as a spice in traditional Indian cuisine.

HISTORY

Ashwagandha has a rich history in Ayurvedic medicine, which has used it for over 3,000 years to promote wellness and longevity. Legend has it that the herb imparts the strength and stamina of a horse, hence its name, which means 'smell of horse' in Sanskrit. They believed this plant provided resistance against disease and stress. Today, ashwagandha continues to be popular for its ability to boost energy, reduce stress and promote overall wellbeing.

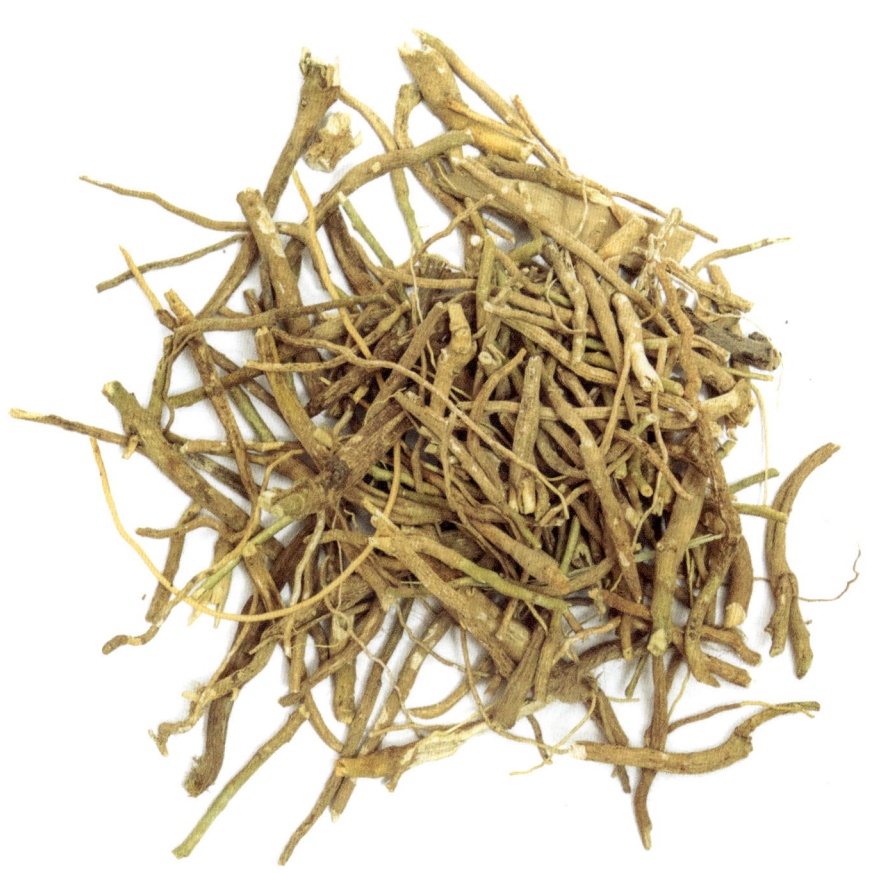

Withania somnifera

anatomē applies ashwagandha to its supplements and oil formulations to promote relaxation, support mood and balance, and enhance libido. These effects are attributed to compounds such as withanolides, which have adaptogenic properties and help the body cope with stress. Ashwagandha also contains compounds like alkaloids and flavonoids with anti-inflammatory and antioxidant properties, making it beneficial for overall health. This herb's ability to balance cortisol levels in the body further aids in reducing stress and anxiety while also boosting energy levels.

Wellbeing challenge: STRESS, LOW LIBIDO
Support ingredient: ASHWAGANDHA

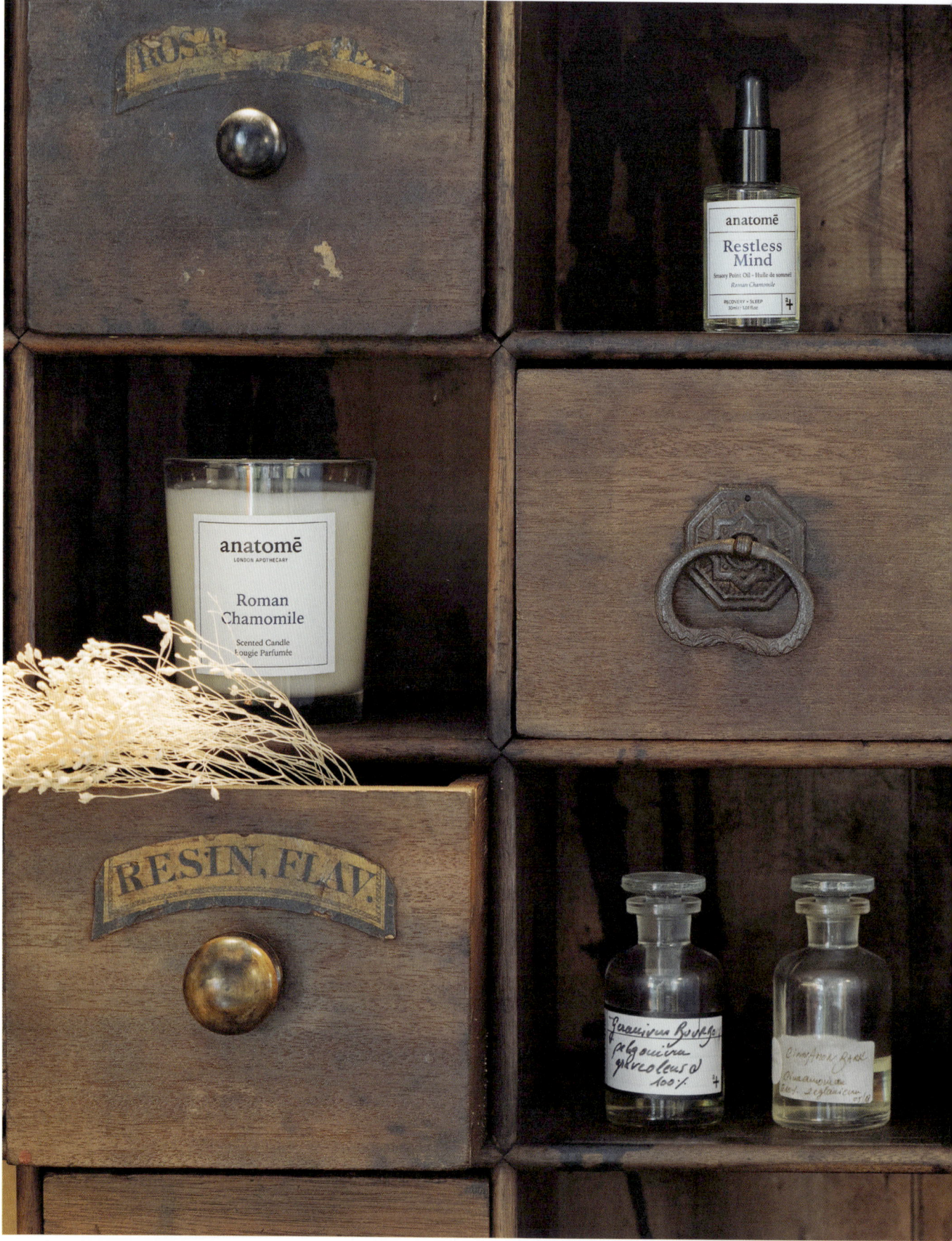

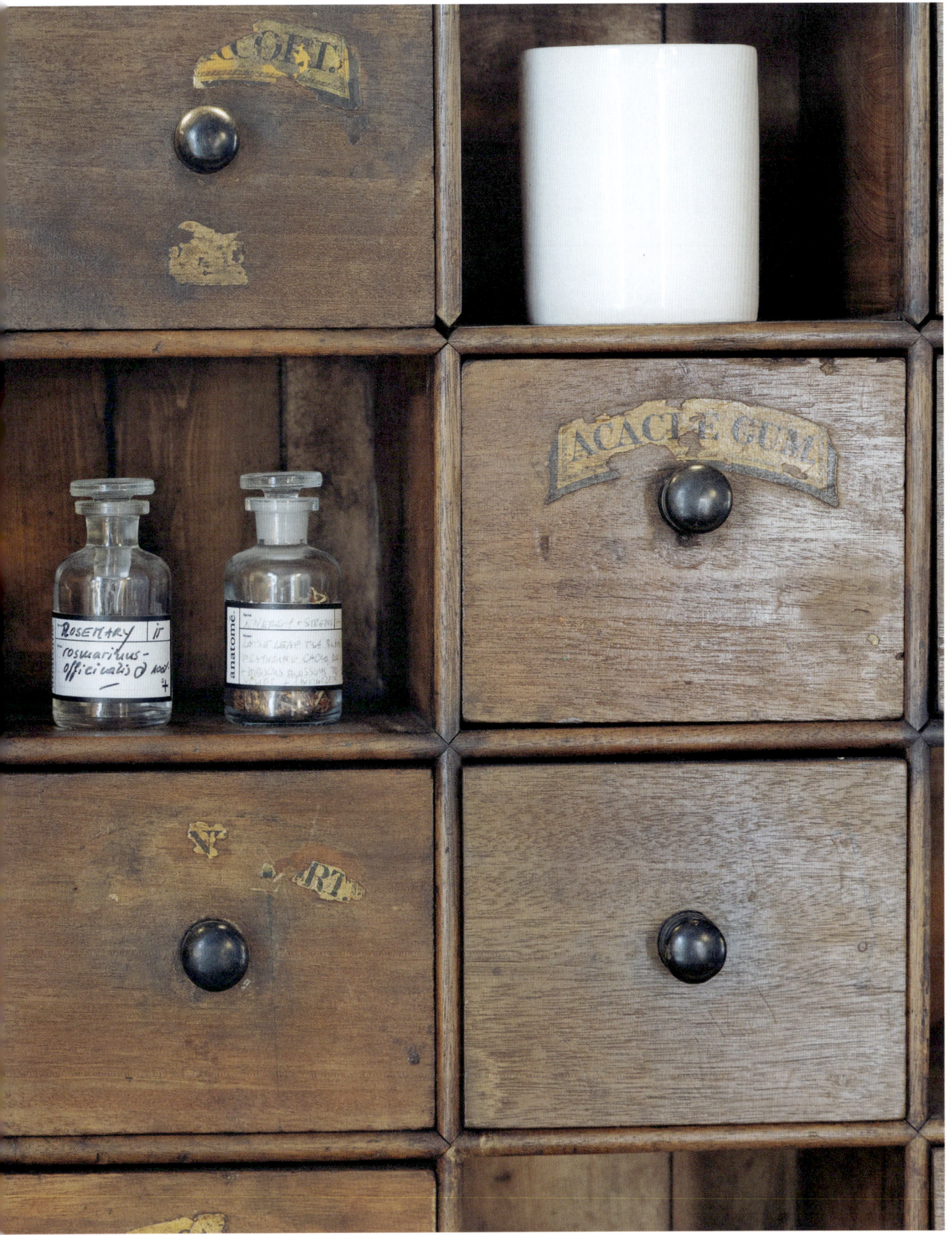

FURTHER READING

Sleep and Health

Why We Sleep by Matthew Walker

The Science of Sleep by Heather Darwall-Smith

Life Time: The New Science of the Body Clock, and How It Can Revolutionize Your Sleep and Health by Russell Foster

Sleepyhead: Narcolepsy, Neuroscience and the Search for a Good Night by Henry Nicholls

Mindfulness and Wellbeing

Ikigai: The Japanese Secret to a Long and Happy Life by Héctor García and Francesc Miralles

Mindfulness: 25 Ways to Live in the Moment Through Art by Christophe Andre and 1 more

The Art of Rest: How to Find Respite in the Modern Age by Claudia Hammond

Plants, Herbs and Medicine

A Curious Herbal by Elizabeth Blackwell

The New Herbal by Leonhart Fuchs

The History of Domestic Plant Medicine by Gabrielle Hatfield

The Apothecaries' Garden by Sue Minter

Aromatica: A Clinical Guide to Essential Oil Therapeutics. Principles and Profiles: 1 by MH Peter Holmes LAc

Ten Drugs: How Plants, Powders, and Pills Have Shaped the History of Medicine by Thomas Hager

Nutrition and Health

Whole: Rethinking the Science of Nutrition by T. Colin Campbell, Ph.D.; Howard Jacobson, Ph.D.

How Not To Die by Michael Greger

Stoicism and Philosophy

How To Be A Stoic: Ancient Wisdom for Modern Living by Massimo Pigliucci

The Daily Stoic: 366 Meditations on Wisdom, Perseverance, and the Art of Living: Featuring new translations of Seneca, Epictetus, and Marcus Aurelius by Ryan Holiday

Exercise and Wellbeing

Yoga: A Manual for Life by Naomi Annand

Caged Lion: Joseph Pilates and His Legacy by John Howard Steel

Scent and Perfume

The Flavour Thesaurus by Niki Segnit

The Secret of Scent: Adventures in Perfume and the Science of Smell by Luca Turin

Perfume: A Century of Scents by Lizzie Ostrom

Essence and Alchemy: A Book of Perfume by Mandy Aftel

Creativity and Self-Discovery

The Poetry Pharmacy: Tried-and-True Prescriptions for the Heart, Mind and Soul by William Sieghart

The Artist's Way: A Spiritual Path to Higher Creativity by Julia Cameron

History and Culture

Past Scents: Historical Perspectives on Smell by Jonathan Reinarz

Karl Blossfeldt. The Complete Published Work by Hans Christian Adam

Why We Swim by Bonnie Tsui

Dioscorides on Pharmacy and Medicine by John M. Riddle

Ancient Egyptian Magic: A Hands-on Guide by Christina Riggs

Nature and Wellbeing

The Healing Magic of Forest Bathing: Finding Calm, Creativity, and Connection in the Natural World by Julia Plevin

INDEX

adaptogens 170
Alcmaeon 59
alcohol 63
Alexander the Great 188, 192
aloe vera 188–9
amino acids 86
Anacharsis 81
anatomē 14, 17, 24
  and aromachology 42
  Cognitive Focus supplement 94
  Essential Oil for Focus 94
  and focus 85
  signifier 35
  sleep formulations 51
  steps for a healthier spine 76
  time management 122
  workplace wellness 110–11
Ancient Egypt 8, 33, 176, 180, 186
Ancient Greece 8, 21, 34, 82, 99, 188
Ancient Rome 21, 81, 180, 188
anxiety 63, 64, 90, 114, 118, 121
  and massage 159
  workplace anxiety 110–11
Apollo 34
apothecaries 29–30
Aristotle 59
aromachology 8, 41–2
Asclepius 34
ashwaganaha 216–17
avocado oil 51, 184–5
awareness meditation 152
Ayurveda 8, 21

back pain 114
balance 14, 47, 62–8
  mood imbalance 62–3
barbital 59
bathrooms 143–5, 149
baths 78
bedrooms 149
  see also sleep
bicycles 82
biosynthesis 170
black pepper 208–9
black spruce 214–15

Blackwell, Elizabeth 22
brain
  cognitive training 93
  and diet 86
  and exercise 83
  and focus 85, 86, 90, 93, 94
  and gut health 96–7
  hormonal imbalances 68
  and sleep 52, 59, 60
breathing 64, 135, 140–1
  4-7-8 breathing technique 141
  abdominal breathing 141
  and meditation 155
  and outdoor living 163
  in the shower 143
Brozler, Anastasia 38
busyness 121, 122
Byron, Lord, vinegar diet 100

camphor 204–5
cardiovascular exercise 74
Chelsea Physic Garden 30
China, meditation 156
chiropractic 23
circadian rhythms 60, 61
cognitive training 93
cold therapy 77
collagen 55
concentration see focus
Cook, Captain James 202
cortisol 50, 51, 170
Covid-19 pandemic 131, 163
cycling 163

dehydration 86
depression 63, 64, 90, 114, 118, 121
  and outdoor living 160
diet 19, 21, 47, 96–105
  and balance 63
  fast eating 117
  and focus 86
  gut health 14, 96–7
  low-fat diets 86
  overeating 117
  steps for a balanced diet 118

through the ages 98–101
  unbalanced 116–18
  vitamins and minerals 86
Donizetti, Gaetano 38
dopamine 63, 159

electroencephalogram (EEG) 60
emotional eating 118
endorphins 73
English peppermint oil 194–5
enteric nervous system (ENS) 96
essential oils 51, 155, 170
eucalyptus 198–201
exercise see movement
eyes, tired 55

Fletcherism 100
focus 14, 47, 85–95
  and diet 86
  and sedentarism 90
  work environment 90, 94
focused attention meditation 152
FOMO (Fear of Missing Out) 108–9, 128
Fonda, Jane 25
food shopping 118
friendships, workplace 111

Galen 59, 81, 99
gastritis 117
geranium bourbon oil 176–7
ginseng 210–11
grapeseed oil 186–7
green cross symbol 34
gut health 14, 96–7, 102–5

Hahnemann, Samuel 22
'halo-effect' improvements 19
herbal medicine 23, 30
Hermes 33
Himalayan and Cornish lavender oil 51
Himalayan salt 192–3
Hippocrates 8, 21, 81
hobbies 67
holistic medicine 24
homeopathy 22

hospital buildings 163
hydrotherapy 23
Hygeia 34
hypnotoxin 60

immune system 159
India, meditation 156
insulin resistance 117

Japanese seaweed 182–3
jojoba oil 190–1
Jouvet, Michel 61

Kellogg, John Harvey 24
ketogenic diet 100
Kneuip, Sebastian 23

Laune, Gideon de 30
lavender oil 51, 172–3
Leonardo da Vinci 8
lion's mane 206–7
lunch breaks 111

massage 159
May Chang oil 174–5
meditation 19, 21, 139, 151–6
Mediterranean diet 99
melatonin 50
mercury 33
metabolic syndrome 117
migraines 159
mindful breathing 64
mindfulness 93, 140, 151
mirrors 143, 145
mood see balance
movement 14, 19, 47, 70–83
    and the brain 83
    cold therapy 77
    exercise and sleep 139
    exercise through the ages 80–1
    gymnasia 81, 83
    health benefits of 70
    recovery time 77
    stretching 76
Murdock, Brendan 37–8, 39, 147
muscle mass 74

Native Americans 190
naturopathy 24
NEAT (non-exercise activity thermogenesis) 74
neck pain 114

neroli 196–7
Nightingale, Florence 163

obesity 100, 114, 117
Olympic Games 82
open monitoring meditation 152
osteopathy 23
outdoor living 160–3

pain 114
peppermint oil 194–5
posture 76, 134
pregnancy 68
primrose oil 212–13
probiotics 105
protein 86

Renaissance 8, 82
Roman chamomile oil 51, 180–1

screen time 114–15
sedentarism 90, 114
self-care 122
Sense of Smell Institute (SSI) 41
serotonin 48, 51, 63, 159
Shakespeare, William 34
showers 143–5
signifiers of wellbeing 33–4
sleep 14, 17, 19, 47, 48–61
    and beauty 55
    and the brain 48, 52, 59, 60
    daytime napping 139
    deep breathing before bed 140
    dreams 50
    and essential oils 51
    and focus 89, 90, 93
    GABA activity 172
    hormones and the nervous system 50
    and the immune system 49
    MSTL (multiple sleep latency test) 61
    positions 56–7
    practice 136–9
        bedtime routine 136
        pre-sleep detox 136
        wake-up time 139
    and recent memory 52
    REM (rapid eye movement) 60, 61
    and screen time 114
    sleep apnoea 90
    sleep through the ages 58–61
snacking 117
snakes 33

social media 25, 86, 101, 108–9, 127, 143
Society of Apothecaries 30, 34
Somali Frankincense oil 51, 178–9
Steiner, Rudolph 24
stress
    adaptogens to support 170
    and balance 64, 67
    and focus 89
    and massage 159
    and outdoor living 160
    and sleep 49, 50, 51, 136
    and workplace anxiety 111

tea tree oil 202–3
terpenes 170
time management 64, 120–2
    smaller tasks 122
    to-do lists 122, 132
Traditional Chinese Medicine 8
Tu Youyou 24

unicorns 34

vagus nerve 135
Velten, Hannah 34
ventilation 163

wakame 182, 183
walking 163
wellbeing 17–91
    assessment of 47
wellbeing practices 125–63
    bathroom practice 143–5
    breathing 135, 140–1
    creating a haven 147–9
    creating a space for 131–2
    posture 134
    sleep 136–9
    time for 128
wellbeing villains 106–23
Wellcome, Henry 34
wellness, concept of 19
windows 163
women's health 22
    hormonal imbalances 68
workplace anxiety 110–11

yoga 136, 151

ACKNOWLEDGEMENTS

A wellness brand is about taking care of others; anatomē was born from a desire to make people feel better. It was built by determined people who employ their talent, passion, dedication and creativity to innovate.

This book is dedicated to those who participated in anatomē – directly and indirectly – since its inception: our families and friends, who supported our ideas and our efforts; anatomē team members, working tirelessly to bring them to life; and our partners, investors and shops around the world who believe in our mission and help us take it across the globe.

We also dedicate this book to all our predecessors in the wellness field: physicians, scientists, aromachologists, philosophers, dietitians, and wellness enthusiasts who took part in the history of feeling better.

ABOUT THE AUTHORS

Brendan Murdock is a creative, designer and entrepreneur with a passion for ingredients and formulations, and the founder of anatomē. His passionate approach to creating potions – for health and pleasure – began not in the lab, but in a restaurant in East London, where he started his career. Later, this fragrance enthusiast delved into the world of grooming with the creation of Murdock London, a brand offering a comprehensive range of products and services for gentlemen's grooming. In 2018, after researching aromachology, botanicals and welllbeing practices, he created anatomē: a brand that champions health and happiness, offering ingredients and proposing ways to practice self-care without the patronising weight of some philosophies in the market – just as Brendan imagined.

Gabriel Weil is a product designer, journalist and creative consultant with a background in fashion and luxury. He has been working with anatomē since 2022, helping shape their tone of voice, create content and develop their storytelling, as well as deliver the brand's message, digitally and physically expanding the modern apothecary vision to communities. When the idea of a book came about, Brendan Murdock asked him to co-write the piece, bringing anatomē to life in print – a medium both are passionate about.

www.anatome.co | @anatomelondon

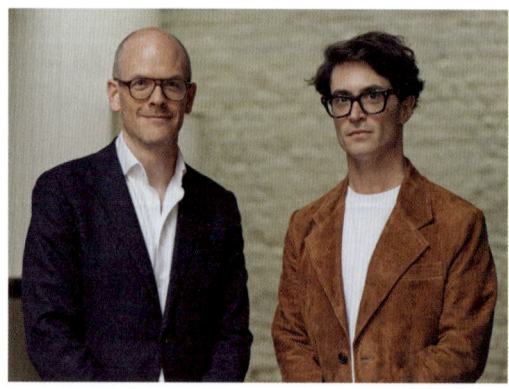